516. 0076 KAL

Accession no.
00949054

PGMC

MRCP1
Pocket Book
1

Cardiology
Haematology
Respiratory Medicine
Rheumatology and Immunology

Third Edition

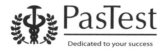

PasTest
Dedicated to your success

JET LIBRARY

MRCP1
Pocket Book
1

Cardiology
Haematology
Respiratory Medicine
Rheumatology and Immunology

Paul Kalra MA MB BChir FRCP
Paul WX Foley MB ChB MRCP (UK)
Keith Patterson FRCP FRCPath
Andres Floto MA PhD MRCP
Anne Barton MSc PhD BSc (Hons) MRCPH

Third Edition

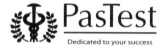

PasTest
Dedicated to your success

© 2008 PASTEST LTD
Egerton Court, Parkgate Estate
Knutsford, Cheshire, WA16 8DX
Telephone: 01565 752000

All rights reserved. No part of this publication may be reproduced, stored in a
retrieval system, or transmitted, in any form or by any means, electronic, mechanical, photocopying, recording or otherwise without the prior permission of the
copyright owner.

Third edition 2008
Second edtion 2004
First edition 2002

ISBN: 1 905635 03 6
ISBN: 978 1 905635 030

A catalogue record for this book is available from the British Library.

The information contained within this book was obtained by the author from
reliable sources. However, while every effort has been made to ensure its accuracy,
no responsibility for loss, damage or injury occasioned to any person acting on
refraining from action as a result of information contained herein can be accepted
by the publishers or author.

PasTest Revision Books and Intensive Courses

PasTest has been established in the field of postgraduate medical
education since 1972, providing revision books and intensive
study courses for doctors preparing for their professional examinations.

Books and courses are available for the following specialties:
**MRCGP, MRCP Parts 1 and 2, MRCPCH Parts 1 and 2, MRCS,
MRCOG Parts 1 and 2, DRCOG, DCH, FRCA, Dentistry.**

For further details contact:
PasTest, Freepost, Knutsford, Cheshire WA16 7BR
Tel: 01565 752000   Fax: 01565 650264
www.pastest.co.uk   enquiries@pastest.co.uk

Text prepared by Keytec Typesetting Ltd, Bridport, Dorset
Printed and bound in the UK by CPI Antony Rowe

CONTENTS

INTRODUCTION

PasTest's MRCP Part 1 Pocket Books are designed to help the busy examination candidate to make the most of every opportunity to revise. With this little book in your pocket, it is the work of a moment to open it, choose a question, decide upon your answers and then check the answer. Revising 'on the run' in this manner is both reassuring (if your answer is correct) and stimulating (if you find any gaps in your knowledge).

The MRCP Part 1 examination consists of two papers, each lasting three hours. Both papers contain 100 'Best of Five' questions (one answer is chosen from five options). Questions in each specialty are randomised across both papers. *No marks are deducted for a wrong answer.*

One-best-answer/'Best of Five' MCQs
An important characteristic of one-best-answer MCQs is that they can be designed to test application of knowledge and clinical problem-solving rather than just the recall of facts. This should change (for the better) the ways in which candidates prepare for MRCP Part 1.

Each one-best MCQ has a question stem, which usually contains clinical information, followed by five branches. All five branches are typically homologous (eg all diagnoses, all laboratory investigations, all antibiotics etc) and should be set out in a logical order (eg alphabetical). Candidates are asked to select the ONE branch that is the best answer to the question. A response is not required to the other four branches. The answer sheet is, therefore, slightly different from that used for true/false MCQs.

A good strategy that can be used with many well-written one-best MCQs is to try to reach the correct answer without first scrutinising the five options. If you can then find the answer you have reached in the option list, then you are probably correct.

One-best-answer MCQs are quicker to answer than multiple true/false MCQs because only one response is needed for each question. Even though the question stem for onebest-answer MCQs is usually longer than for true/false questions, and therefore takes a little longer to read carefully, it is reasonable to set more one-best than true/false MCQs for the same exam duration – in this instance 60 true/false and 100 one-best are used in exams of 2 hours' duration.

Application of Knowledge and Clinical Problem-Solving
Unlike true/false MCQs, which test mainly the recall of knowledge, one-best-answer questions test application and problem-solving. This makes them more effective test items and is one of the reasons why testing time can be reduced. In

order to answer these questions correctly, it is necessary to apply basic knowledge – not just the ability to remember it. Furthermore, candidates who cannot reach the correct answer by applying their knowledge are much less likely to be able to choose the right answer by guessing than they were with true/false MCQs. This gives a big advantage to the best candidates, who have good knowledge and can apply it in clinical situations.

Books like the ones in this series, which consist of 'Best of Five' questions in subject categories, can help you to focus on specific topics and to isolate your weaknesses. You should plan a revision timetable to help you spread your time evenly over the range of subjects likely to appear in the examination. PasTest's **Essential Revision Notes for MRCP** by P Kalra will provide you with essential notes on all aspects of the syllabus.

THIRD EDITION

Cardiology
Paul Kalra MA MB BChir FRCP, Consultant Cardiologist, Portsmouth Hospitals NHS Trust.
Paul WX Foley MB ChB MRCP (UK), Specialist Registrar in Cardiology and Honorary Research Fellow at the University of Birmingham

Haematology
Keith Patterson FRCP FRCPath, Consultant Haematologist, University College, London Hospital, London.

Respiratory Medicine
Andres Floto MA PhD MRCP Wellcome Trust Senior Fellow, Cambridge Institute for Medical Research, University of Cambridge and Consultant, Cystic Fibrosis/Lung Defence Unit, Papworth Hospital, Cambridge.

Rheumatology and Immunology
Anne Barton MSc PhD BSc(Hons) MRCP, Consultant Rheumatologist and Clinical Lecturer, East Cheshire NHS Trust and University of Manchester.

SECOND EDITION

Cardiology
Paul Kalra MRCP, Consultant Cardiologist, Portsmouth Hospitals NHS Trust.
John Paisey BM MRCP, SpR and Research Fellow, Wessex Cardiothoracic Unit, Southampton General Hospital, Southampton.

Haematology
Keith Patterson FRCP FRCPath, Consultant Haematologist, University College London Hospital, London.
Mary Frances McMullin MD FRCP (Edin) FRCPath FRCPI, PGCHET, Reader Consultant Haematologist, Department of Haematology, Queen's University, Belfast City Hospital, Belfast.

Respiratory Medicine
Howard Branley MB ChB MSc MRCP, Raynaud's and Scleroderma Association Research Fellow, National Heart and Lung Institute, royal Brompton and the Hammersmith Hospitals, London.

Rheumatology – Pocket Book 4
Anne Barton MSc PhD BSc(Hons) MRCP, Consultant Rheumatologist and Clinical Lecturer, East Cheshire NHS Trust and University of Manchester.

Alan J Hakim MA MRCP, Consultant Rheumatologist and General Physician, Whipp's Cross University Hospital, London, Honorary Consultant Rheumatologist, University College London Hsopitals.

Immunology – Pocket Book 4

Neil Snowden FRCP FRCPath Consultant Rheumatologist, North Manchester General Hospital Manchester.

Alan J Hakim MA MRCP, Consultant Rheumatologist and General Physician, Whipp's Cross University Hospital, London, Honorary Consultant Rheumatologist, University College London Hsopitals.

Cardiology

Best of Five

Questions

CARDIOLOGY 'BEST OF FIVE' QUESTIONS

For each of the questions select the ONE most appropriate answer from the options provided.

1.1 A 78-year-old man receives a VVIR pacemaker for complete heart block with profound hypotension. At 3-month review in the Out-Patients Department (OPD) he feels well, but cannon waves are noted in the internal jugular vein. Which is the most likely cause?

☐ **A** Atrial flutter

☐ **B** Pacemaker failure

☐ **C** Pericardial effusion

☐ **D** Ventricular tachycardia (VT)

☐ **E** VVI pacing

1.2 A 50-year-old man is hypertensive with repeated blood pressure recordings of >160/95 mmHg. He is already taking a thiazide diuretic as well as aspirin 75 mg and a statin. There are no apparent secondary causes of hypertension. He has previously undergone coronary artery bypass grafting. Which one of the following is the most appropriate add on antihypertensive treatment?

☐ **A** α-Blocker

☐ **B** Angiotensin-converting enzyme (ACE) inhibitor

☐ **C** Angiotensin receptor blocker

☐ **D** β-Blocker

☐ **E** Calcium-channel antagonist

1.3 A patient presents with severe intra-scapular pain. Computed tomography (CT) scan confirms a diagnosis of type B aortic dissection. Clinical examination reveals sinus tachycardia of 100 bpm and blood pressure 150/84 mmHg (similar in both arms). Which one of the following is the most appropriate immediate intervention?

☐ **A** Intravenous β-blocker

☐ **B** Intravenous glyceryl trinitrate (GTN)

☐ **C** Oral angiotensin-converting enzyme (ACE) inhibitor

☐ **D** Referral for urgent surgery

☐ **E** Trans-oesophageal echo

1.4 A 50-year-old man is found collapsed in the medical admissions unit. He is unresponsive. There are no signs of life. Which of the following is the correct next action?

☐ **A** Call for help

☐ **B** Commence cardiopulmonary resuscitation (CPR)

☐ **C** Connect up defibrillator to monitor rhythm

☐ **D** Precordial thump

☐ **E** Two rescue breaths

1.5 Once monitoring is attached at a cardiac arrest the patient is found to be in ventricular fibrillation. He is receiving basic life support. What is the correct next action?

☐ **A** Intravenous adrenaline

☐ **B** Intravenous sodium bicarbonate

☐ **C** Intubate the patient

☐ **D** 150 J monophasic shock

☐ **E** 150 J biphasic shock

1.6 A 53-year-old woman with prior anterior myocardial infarction (MI) and moderate left ventricular function on trans-thoracic echocardiography complains of dyspnoea on exertion (New York Heart Association (NYHA) Class II). Coronary angiography reveals an occluded left anterior descending artery, but otherwise patent vessels. Cardiac magnetic resonance scanning reveals scarring in the anterior wall with no viable tissue. Current medications include aspirin 75 mg, ramipril 5 mg bd, simvastatin 40 mg od. She cannot tolerate β-blockers due to severe asthma. She is in sinus rhythm with blood pressure 110/60 mmHg and creatinine 140 mmol/l. What additional treatment should be considered?

☐ **A** Amiodarone

☐ **B** Candesartan

☐ **C** Digoxin

☐ **D** Eplerenone

☐ **E** Spironolactone

    Answers on pages 73–91

1.7 **A 40-year-old man presents with a 3-hour history of chest pain to a minor injuries unit, and his electrocardiogram (ECG) shows sinus rhythm with anterior ST elevation. He has received 300 mg aspirin. His myocardial infarction should be treated as follows:**

☐ **A** Clopidogrel 300 mg and streptokinase infusion

☐ **B** Clopidogrel 300 mg and tenecteplase

☐ **C** Clopidogrel 600 mg and transfer for primary percutaneous coronary intervention (travelling time to centre 1 hour)

☐ **D** Streptokinase infusion

☐ **E** Tenecteplase followed by enoxaparin 1 mg/kg

1.8 **A 70-year-old man presents with a 2-year history of exertional dyspnoea and episodic syncope. The patient has recently moved to the area. While he himself is unaware of any significant past medical history he has been receiving regular (annual) haematology follow-up. He takes no regular medication. Examination reveals sinus rhythm and a blood pressure of 90/60 mmHg. The electrocardiogram (ECG) shows small complexes and the cardio-thoracic ratio is less than 50%. An echocardiogram is reported as showing left ventricular hypertrophy, a normal cavity size and impaired left ventricular function with failure of systolic myocardial thickening. What is the most likely diagnosis?**

☐ **A** Cardiac amyloidosis

☐ **B** Cardiac lymphoma

☐ **C** Coronary artery disease

☐ **D** Haemochromatosis

☐ **E** Hypertrophic cardiomyopathy

1.9 A 47-year-old man with dilated cardiomyopathy presumable secondary to myocarditis 5 years previously re-presents with increasing symptoms. He is now dyspnoeic on climbing stairs and taking a shower. His ECG shows sinus rhythm with a PR interval of 220 ms and left bundle branch block (QRS duration of 160 ms). Clinically he is euvolaemic, with a blood pressure of 80/50 mmHg. His medication is carvedilol 50 mg bd, ramipril 5 mg bd, furosemide 40 mg od. The next therapy is:

☐ **A** Cardiac resynchronisation pacemaker

☐ **B** Cardiac transplantation

☐ **C** Dual chamber pacemaker

☐ **D** Implantable cardioverter defibrillator

☐ **E** Left ventricular assist device

1.10 A 45-year-old man has an anterior myocardial infarction treated by primary percutaneous coronary intervention (PCI) to the left anterior descending artery (LAD). He remains in pulmonary oedema on day three of his admission. His blood pressure is 100/60 mmHg, heart rate 70 bpm (sinus rhythm), and he is passing good volumes of urine. His creatinine is 100 mmol/l, potassium 4.5 mmol/l. His medication includes aspirin 75 mg, clopidogrel 75 mg od, and simvastatin 40 mg od, iv furosemide 80 mg bd and intravenous GTN. Which of the following should now be added?

☐ **A** Bisoprolol 1.25 mg od

☐ **B** Ramipril 1.25 mg od + start bisoprolol 1.25 mg od

☐ **C** Oral nitrate

☐ **D** Ramipril 1.25 mg bd

☐ **E** Ramipril 1.25 mg bd + eplerenone 25 mg od

Answers on pages 73–91

1.11 **A 60-year-old man who is awaiting aortic valve replacement (AVR) surgery for severe aortic stenosis is admitted in biventricular heart failure and cardiogenic shock. Coronary angiography previously showed unobstructed coronaries. Left ventricular (LV) function at trans-thoracic echocardiography was poor, blood pressure (BP) 100/60 mmHg. His creatinine is now 160 mmol/l (previously 100). The next step should be:**

- ☐ **A** Intubation and ventilation
- ☐ **B** Intravenous fluids to correct hypotension
- ☐ **C** Inotropes
- ☐ **D** Intra-aortic balloon pump insertion
- ☐ **E** Intra-aortic balloon pump insertion and trial of sodium nitroprusside

1.12 **A 36-year-old woman is admitted with severe central chest pain in association with anterior ST elevation. Her blood pressure is 70/40 mmHg, pulse 110 bpm (sinus rhythm). She has received aspirin 300 mg. Her management should be:**

- ☐ **A** Clopidogrel 600 mg + primary percutaneous coronary intervention + intra-aortic balloon pump insertion
- ☐ **B** Immediate thrombolysis with reteplase + clopidogrel 75 mg
- ☐ **C** Clopidogrel 75 mg + primary PCI
- ☐ **D** Immediate thrombolysis with reteplase + clopidogrel 300 mg
- ☐ **E** Immediate thrombolysis with reteplase + clopidogrel 600 mg

1.13 **A 30-year-old man presents with ventricular tachycardia (VT) with left bundle branch block (LBBB) morphology that reverts to sinus rhythm (SR). There is a family history of sudden death. His electrocardiogram (ECG) shows SR with partial right bundle branch block (RBBB) and T-wave inversion in V1 to V3. The QT is normal. His echocardiogram shows good left ventricular function, but the right ventricle is dilated. Confirmatory diagnosis may be obtained by:**

- ☐ **A** Cardiac magnetic resonance imaging
- ☐ **B** Coronary angiography
- ☐ **C** Computed tomography (CT) pulmonary angiography
- ☐ **D** Genetic testing
- ☐ **E** Lung perfusion imaging

1.14 A 60-year-old man presents with a 3-month history of increasing exertional dyspnoea and ankle oedema. His ECG shows atrial flutter with a ventricular rate of 150 bpm. Enoxaparin 1.5 mg/kg od is started. The optimal treatment is:

- ☐ **A** DC cardioversion
- ☐ **B** Digoxin
- ☐ **C** Amiodarone iv
- ☐ **D** Amiodarone and digoxin oral
- ☐ **E** Trans-oesophageal echocardiography, and if satisfactory proceed to DC cardioversion

1.15 A 35-year-old man is referred because his electrocardiogram (ECG) shows left ventricular hypertrophy. He has previously had a stroke and has renal failure. Examination reveals a long-standing rash in a bathing trunk distribution. The most likely diagnosis is:

- ☐ **A** Anderson–Fabry disease
- ☐ **B** Burgada syndrome
- ☐ **C** Coarctation of the aorta
- ☐ **D** Hypertensive cardiomyopathy
- ☐ **E** Hypertrophic cardiomyopathy

1.16 A 70-year-old woman is admitted with recurrent syncope. She has been treated for paroxysmal atrial fibrillation with amiodarone and warfarin. Her ECG shows sinus bradycardia, rate 50 bpm, PR interval 150 ms, QT interval 480 ms, QTc 500 ms. While attached to a monitor she is syncopal and self-terminating torsades de pointes is noted. Serum potassium is 5.0 mmol/l. What is the most appropriate next step?

- ☐ **A** Check serum magnesium levels
- ☐ **B** Intravenous amiodarone
- ☐ **C** Intravenous calcium chloride
- ☐ **D** Intravenous lidocaine
- ☐ **E** Temporary pacing

Answers on pages 73–91

1.17   A 45-year-old man has a dual chamber pacemaker inserted for complete heart block. He represents with a stroke 3 months later. Interrogation of the pacemaker shows sinus rhythm with no evidence of atrial fibrillation. A routine ECG shows atrial and ventricular pacing, and the ventricular depolarisation has a right bundle branch pattern. The most likely cause of the stroke is:

- ☐ **A**   Coronary sinus pacing
- ☐ **B**   Fractured pacing lead
- ☐ **C**   Inadvertent left ventricular pacing
- ☐ **D**   Subclavian vein thrombosis
- ☐ **E**   Tricuspid valve endocarditis

1.18   A 42-year-old man who previously underwent aortic valve replacement for infective endocarditis is admitted with general malaise and fever. Blood cultures grow enterococcus and he is started on appropriate antibiotics. A trans-oesophageal echocardiogram on admission shows a normally functioning prosthetic aortic valve. Serial C-reactive protein levels show a drop from 200 to 30 mg/l with treatment over 3 weeks. His electrocardiogram (ECG) shows sinus rhythm and a lengthening PR interval from 150 on admission to 250 ms. The next appropriate procedure is:

- ☐ **A**   Dual chamber pacemaker
- ☐ **B**   Radiolabelled white cell scan
- ☐ **C**   Single chamber (ventricular) pacemaker
- ☐ **D**   Trans-oesophageal echocardiogram
- ☐ **E**   Trans-thoracic echocardiogram

1.19   An 80-year-old woman is admitted with cardiac failure and atrial fibrillation with a rapid ventricular response. A chest radiograph shows cardiomegaly and pulmonary oedema. The most appropriate oral medication to treat the atrial fibrillation is:

- ☐ **A**   Amiodarone
- ☐ **B**   Atenolol
- ☐ **C**   Digoxin
- ☐ **D**   Flecainide
- ☐ **E**   Verapamil

1.20 A 35-year-old man is troubled with severe limiting paroxysmal atrial fibrillation despite multiple anti-arrhythmics including flecainide, bisoprolol, and propafenone. An echocardiogram shows the heart is normal in structure and function. Which would be the best option now?

- ☐ **A** Ablate the arteriovenous (AV) node and insert a pacemaker (ablate and pace)
- ☐ **B** Amiodarone
- ☐ **C** Atrial fibrillation surgery
- ☐ **D** Implantable atrial defibrillator
- ☐ **E** Radiofrequency atrial fibrillation ablation

1.21 A 70-year-old woman undergoes a mitral valve replacement for severe mitral regurgitation. Pre-operative evaluation reveals good left and right ventricular function with normal pulmonary pressure, and unobstructed coronary arteries. Six hours post-operatively she becomes hypotensive and tachycardic. The central venous pressure (CVP) has increased from 5 to 20 cm. Clinical examination reveals a clear chest and normal prosthetic heart sounds. The most likely diagnosis is

- ☐ **A** Constriction
- ☐ **B** Gastro-intestinal bleed
- ☐ **C** Pericardial tamponade
- ☐ **D** Pulmonary embolism
- ☐ **E** Right ventricular infarction

1.22 A 20-year-old women is diagnosed with Marfan's syndrome. Her blood pressure is 130/80 mmHg. A magnetic resonance aortogram measures the greatest width of the aorta at 3.8 cm. Treatment should be started with:

- ☐ **A** Bisoprolol
- ☐ **B** Methyldopa
- ☐ **C** No treatment
- ☐ **D** Ramipril
- ☐ **E** Sotalol

1.23 A 50-year-old woman undergoes primary PCI for an acute inferior myocardial infarction. She has episodes of atrial fibrillation, which are treated with oral amiodarone. Initially she is haemodynamically stable, but 2 days later she has a cardiac arrest and is found to be in ventricular fibrillation, which is successfully defibrillated. The most likely cause of the arrest is:

☐ **A** Acute stent thrombosis

☐ **B** Hypovolaemia

☐ **C** Idiopathic ventricular fibrillation

☐ **D** Left ventricular scarring

☐ **E** Peri-infarct arrhythmia

1.24 A 60-year-old man presents with two episodes of syncope over the past 2 months, which occurred while resting. He is not taking any medications. A resting electrocardiogram (ECG) shows sinus rhythm with bifascicular block and a 24-hour tape is unremarkable. The most sensible next step is:

☐ **A** Carotid sinus massage

☐ **B** Electrophysiological study

☐ **C** Exercise stress test

☐ **D** Implantable loop recorder insertion

☐ **E** Tilt test

1.25 A 65-year-old man presents with recurrent acute pulmonary oedema without chest pain. His electrocardiogram (ECG) is normal. An echocardiogram shows preserved systolic function, moderate left ventricular hypertrophy and normal valvular function. Coronary angiography shows unobstructed arteries. His creatinine is elevated at 150 mmol/l. Renal ultrasound reveals the left kidney is 9 cm and the right is 11 cm. He has a right femoral bruit. What is the next investigation of choice?

☐ **A** Computed tomography (CT) pulmonary angiogram

☐ **B** Magnetic resonance (MR) renal angiogram

☐ **C** Renal biopsy

☐ **D** Implantation of loop recorder (Reveal™ device)

☐ **E** Twenty-four hour urine collection for catecholamines

1.26 A 16-year-old Thai boy is admitted with a syncopal episode. His brother died at the age of 6 from unexplained sudden death and a post mortem was completely normal. Resting electrocardiogram (ECG) and echocardiography are normal. The next appropriate investigation is:

☐ **A** Carotid sinus massage

☐ **B** Cardiac magnetic resonance imaging (CMR)

☐ **C** Coronary angiography

☐ **D** Flecainide challenge

☐ **E** Tilt test

1.27 A 54-year-old man is admitted with chest pain and ST elevation in the inferior limb leads. He is thrombolysed with streptokinase. In the next 6 hours his blood pressure is 90/40 mmHg with poor urine output. A central venous line and Swan–Ganz catheter are inserted. His CVP is 15 cmH$_2$O and pulmonary capillary wedge pressure (PCWP) is 20 mmH$_2$O. What is the optimal definitive treatment?

☐ **A** Inotropic support

☐ **B** Intravenous furosemide (frusemide)

☐ **C** Fluid challenge

☐ **D** Repeat thrombolysis

☐ **E** Rescue angioplasty

1.28 A 35-year-old patient who has recently arrived from the Indian subcontinent presents with rapid onset of shortness of breath on exertion having previously been well. Examination reveal an irregular pulse with an apical rate of 120 bpm. An echocardiogram shows significant mitral stenosis. What is the most likely cause of the deterioration?

☐ **A** Bacterial endocarditis

☐ **B** Concomitant ischaemic heart disease

☐ **C** Development of atrial fibrillation

☐ **D** Rapid progression of mitral valve disease

☐ **E** Recurrence of rheumatic fever

Answers on pages 73–91

1.29 A 58-year-old man who is taking no medication is referred to the Out-Patient's Department with palpitations. He has a history of previous anterior myocardial infarction and an echocardiogram reveals moderately impaired left ventricular function. An ambulatory monitor shows frequent symptomatic episodes of intermittent atrial fibrillation. Which one of the following combinations would be the most appropriate initial treatment?

☐ **A** Amiodarone and aspirin

☐ **B** Bisoprolol and warfarin

☐ **C** Digoxin and warfarin

☐ **D** Flecainide and warfarin

☐ **E** Sotalol and aspirin

1.30 A 45-year-old man presents with an episode of central chest pain lasting for one hour. He is a current smoker with a strong family history of premature coronary artery disease. His resting electrocardiogram (ECG) is normal. Which one of these investigations would be the most helpful in assisting with planning initial management?

☐ **A** Angiogram

☐ **B** Echocardiogram

☐ **C** Exercise test

☐ **D** Troponin I level

☐ **E** Ventilation/perfusion scan

1.31 A 70-year-old woman presents with severe chest pain and nausea. Examination reveals a pulse rate of 40 bpm, blood pressure 100/60 mmHg and clear lung fields. Her electrocardiogram (ECG) confirms significant inferior ST-segment elevation with complete heart block (CHB). She has received 300 mg of oral aspirin. Which one of the following would be the optimal therapeutic intervention?

☐ **A** Dobutamine infusion

☐ **B** External pacing

☐ **C** Primary percutaneous coronary intervention with temporary wire cover

☐ **D** Temporary pacing-wire insertion

☐ **E** Thrombolysis with streptokinase

1.32 A 72-year-old man complains of limiting exertional chest tightness. He has clinical evidence of significant aortic stenosis and left ventricular hypertrophy on the resting ECG. Trans-thoracic echocardiography demonstrates a peak aortic valve gradient of 50 mmHg with moderate left ventricular function. Cardiac catheterisation is planned. What would be the most helpful information to obtain from this investigation?

☐ **A** Aortic valve gradient

☐ **B** Left ventricular function

☐ **C** Presence of co-existing coronary artery disease

☐ **D** Right heart pressures

☐ **E** Severity of co-existing aortic incompetence

1.33 A patient with dilated cardiomyopathy and permanent atrial fibrillation (AF) has a resting heart rate of 110 bpm. Twenty-four hour taped recordings show even higher uncontrolled rates, particularly associated with exercise. He is already taking 187.5 mg of digoxin and has a normal creatinine. Which one of the following would be the most beneficial treatment?

☐ **A** Addition of β-blocker

☐ **B** Addition of verapamil

☐ **C** Arteriovenous (AV) node ablation and permanent pacemaker insertion

☐ **D** DC cardioversion

☐ **E** Increase digoxin to 250 mg

1.34 A 30-year-old window cleaner has a 1-year history of frequent, rapid, palpitations associated with dizziness, but no actual syncope. He drinks approximately 35 units of alcohol per week but is on no regular medication. His resting electrocardiogram (ECG) confirms a diagnosis of Wolff–Parkinson–White syndrome (WPW). Which one of the following is the most appropriate treatment?

☐ **A** Amiodarone

☐ **B** Flecainide

☐ **C** Radiofrequency ablation of the accessory pathway

☐ **D** Radiofrequency modification of the arteriovenous (AV) node

☐ **E** Sotalol

Answers on pages 73–91

1.35 A 60-year-old woman presents with increasing swelling of the ankles, abdominal distension and dyspnoea. She has a past medical history of pulmonary tuberculosis as a child and a left mastectomy and subsequent radiotherapy 5 years previously. On examination she is apyrexial, with a sinus tachycardia of 100 bpm and blood pressure of 110/60 mmHg (paradox 8 mmHg). She has significant peripheral oedema and ascites. Her jugular venous pressure (JPV) is elevated at 8 cm above the sternal angle and demonstrates a rapid y-descent. What is the most likely diagnosis?

- ☐ **A** Cardiac tamponade
- ☐ **B** Constrictive pericarditis
- ☐ **C** Intra-abdominal neoplasm
- ☐ **D** Severe tricuspid incompetence
- ☐ **E** Superior vena cava obstruction

1.36 The following findings are obtained during right and left heart catheterisation in a 50-year-old woman. Pressures (mmHg): right atrial = mean 9; right ventricle = 35/2; pulmonary artery = 36/14; pulmonary capillary wedge = mean 10; aorta = 120/65. Saturations (%): superior vena cava = 65; right atrial = 76; right ventricle = 77; pulmonary artery = 75; aorta = 97. She has no significant past medical history, except recent onset of paroxysmal atrial flutter. What is the most likely diagnosis?

- ☐ **A** Atrial septal defect (ASD)–ostium primum
- ☐ **B** ASD–ostium secundum
- ☐ **C** Sinus venosus defect
- ☐ **D** Tricuspid incompetence
- ☐ **E** Ventricular septal defect (VSD)

1.37 An asymptomatic 45-year-old man has a systolic murmur. He is in sinus rhythm. Trans-thoracic echocardiography demonstrates normal left ventricular function and dimensions, together with moderate mitral regurgitation secondary to posterior mitral valve leaflet prolapse. The left atrium is mildly enlarged at 4.4 cm. The right ventricular systolic pressure at echocardiography is estimated at 50 mmHg. Which one of the following is the most appropriate course of action?

- ☐ **A** Amiodarone to maintain sinus rhythm
- ☐ **B** Recommend bacterial endocarditis prophylaxis and discharge
- ☐ **C** Regular clinical follow-up with repeat echocardiography
- ☐ **D** Regular clinical follow-up with repeat echocardiography and anticoagulation with warfarin
- ☐ **E** Trans-oesophageal echo and early referral for mitral valve replacement

1.38 Day 2 after an anterior MI, a 60-year-old man develops cardiogenic shock with blood pressure of 80/50 mmHg and oliguria. A Swan–Ganz catheter is inserted and reveals a pulmonary capillary wedge pressure (PCWP) of 20 mmHg; systemic vascular resistance (SVR) 1580 (normal: 900–1200 dyne.s/cm^2) and cardiac index (CI) of 1.8 (cardiac output/body surface area, normal: 2.8–3.5 l/min per m^2). Which one of the following would be the most appropriate initial treatment?

- ☐ **A** Dobutamine
- ☐ **B** Dopamine
- ☐ **C** Intravenous GTN
- ☐ **D** Intravenous fluids (gentle)
- ☐ **E** Noradrenaline (norepinephrine)

Answers on pages 73–91

1.39 A patient has a pulmonary embolus, proved by spiral computed tomography (CT) scanning. Twenty-four hours after initiation of low-molecular-weight heparin (LMWH) therapy, he becomes hypotensive, tachycardic and hypoxic, without evidence of acute bleeding. His JVP is elevated at 8 cm above the sternal notch. Which one of the following would be the desired intervention?

☐ **A** Change LMWH to intravenous unfractionated heparin

☐ **B** Inotropic support

☐ **C** Insertion of an inferior vena cava filter

☐ **D** Thrombolysis with streptokinase

☐ **E** Thrombolysis with tissue plasminogen activator

1.40 Six months after prosthetic mitral valve replacement a patient presents with a 2-month history of rigors, anorexia, fatigue and weight loss. The C-reactive protein (CRP) is elevated at 110 mg/l. Trans-thoracic echo confirms moderate paravalvular regurgitation with vegetation. Which one of the following is the most likely infecting organism?

☐ **A** *Candida albicans*

☐ **B** *Escherichia coli*

☐ **C** *Staphylococcus aureus*

☐ **D** *Staphylococcus epidermidis*

☐ **E** *Streptococcus viridans*

1.41 A 40-year-old male smoker is found to have a fasting cholesterol of 8.0 mmol/l and triglycerides of 1.8 mmol/l. He is hypertensive with a strong family history of premature coronary artery disease. Which one of the following would be the recommended intervention?

☐ **A** Cholestyramine

☐ **B** Diet

☐ **C** Ezetimibe

☐ **D** Omega-3 fish oils

☐ **E** Simvastatin

1.42 A patient with previous history of myocardial infarction presents with a broad-complex tachycardia. Blood pressure is 110/60 mmHg. Lung fields are clear. What is the most appropriate initial management therapy?

- ☐ **A** Intravenous digoxin
- ☐ **B** Intravenous amiodarone
- ☐ **C** Oral amiodarone
- ☐ **D** Overdrive pacing
- ☐ **E** Trans-oesophageal echo and DC cardioversion if no thrombus

1.43 A patient undergoes assessment for suitability for percutaneous trans-septal mitral valvuloplasty for the treatment of rheumatic mitral stenosis. The presence of which one of the following features would most likely preclude this form of intervention?

- ☐ **A** Atrial fibrillation
- ☐ **B** Coronary artery disease
- ☐ **C** Mild mitral regurgitation
- ☐ **D** Pulmonary hypertension
- ☐ **E** Thrombus in the left atrial appendage

1.44 An asymptomatic 30-year-old gym instructor has a routine medical examination. An electrocardiogram (ECG) demonstrates left bundle branch block (LBBB). Which one of the following clinical signs is most likely to be present?

- ☐ **A** Displaced apex beat
- ☐ **B** Fourth heart sound
- ☐ **C** Left ventricular heave
- ☐ **D** Reverse splitting of the second heart sound
- ☐ **E** Third heart sound

Answers on pages 73–91

1.45   A 15-year-old refugee presents with a short history of fever, malaise and
        flitting polyarthritis. Clinical examination reveals a soft apical systolic
        murmur and pericardial rub. Investigations demonstrate elevated
        inflammatory markers (CRP and ESR). Which one of the following is the
        most likely diagnosis?

   ☐   **A**   Acute rheumatic fever
   ☐   **B**   Atrial myxoma
   ☐   **C**   Kawasaki disease
   ☐   **D**   Subacute bacterial endocarditis (SBE)
   ☐   **E**   Systemic lupus erythematosus

1.46   A patient undergoes successful elective DC cardioversion for lone AF.
        Before the cardioversion he is taking warfarin, amiodarone and
        bisoprolol. Which one of the following drug combinations would be
        preferred before out-patient review in three months?

   ☐   **A**   Amiodarone and aspirin
   ☐   **B**   Amiodarone and warfarin
   ☐   **C**   Bisoprolol and aspirin
   ☐   **D**   Bisoprolol and warfarin
   ☐   **E**   Warfarin alone

1.47   A 40-year-old man is investigated after having undergone successful
        community resuscitation following an episode of ventricular fibrillation.
        Echocardiogram demonstrates no structural abnormalities and coronary
        arteries are normal at angiography. Which one of the following would be
        the most appropriate long-term management?

   ☐   **A**   Amiodarone
   ☐   **B**   Implantable cardioverter defibrillator
   ☐   **C**   Procainamide
   ☐   **D**   Sotalol
   ☐   **E**   VT stimulation study and ablation

1.48 When contemplating coronary artery bypass grafting, which one of the following is the preferred option for revascularising the left anterior descending artery (LAD)?

☐ **A** Direct endarterectomy

☐ **B** Left internal mammary artery

☐ **C** Radial artery

☐ **D** Right internal mammary artery

☐ **E** Saphenous vein graft

1.49 A 30-year-old man presents with recurrent episodes of chest pain and exertional pre-syncope. There is a family history of sudden death. Resting electrocardiogram (ECG) demonstrates features of left ventricular hypertrophy (LVH) and precordial T-wave inversion. Which one of the following is the most likely diagnosis?

☐ **A** Dilated cardiomyopathy

☐ **B** Hypertrophic cardiomyopathy

☐ **C** Ischaemic heart disease

☐ **D** Pulmonary embolic disease

☐ **E** Supra-valvular aortic stenosis

1.50 An infant with trisomy 21 (Down's syndrome) presents with failure to gain weight and clinical evidence of heart failure. Which one of the following congenital cardiac abnormalities is most likely to account for this?

☐ **A** Aortic incompetence

☐ **B** Endocardial cushion defect

☐ **C** Mitral valve prolapse

☐ **D** Pulmonary hypertension

☐ **E** Secundum ASD

Haematology

Best of Five

Questions

HAEMATOLOGY 'BEST OF FIVE' QUESTIONS

For each of the questions select the ONE most appropriate answer from the options provided.

2.1 One week after delivery of twins by Caesarean section, a 35-year-old woman is referred to the Maternity Unit with a pyrexia of unknown origin (PUO). On examination, she appears slightly confused and has temperature of 38.5 °C, blood pressure (BP) 160/75 mmHg, pulse 106 reg. A blood count and blood cultures are performed:

	WBC × 10^9/l	RBC × 10^{12}/l	Hb g/dl	Hct ratio	MCV Fl	MCH pg	MCHC g/dl	RDW	Plt × 10^9/l
Blood count									
	4–11	M 4.7–6.1; F 4.2–5.4	M 13–17.5; F 12–16	M 0.42–0.50; F 0.37–0.47	80–99	27–31	32–35	11.5–14.5	150–400
Blood cultures									
	16.9	3.19	9.6	0.313	98	30.1	30.6	17.0	14

Automated differential: neutrophils 78%, lymphocytes 19%, monocytes 2%, eosinophils 1%. Erythrocyte sedimentation rate (ESR) 35 mm/h. Which of the following would provide strongest supporting evidence for a diagnosis of thrombotic thrombocytopenic purpura?

- ☐ **A** Elevated reticulocyte count
- ☐ **B** Increased megakaryocytes in marrow aspirate
- ☐ **C** Serum lactate dehydrogenase (LDH) level of 1500 (normal 100–300 IU/l)
- ☐ **D** Prolonged prothrombin time
- ☐ **E** HLA (human leucocyte antigen) alloantibodies in serum

2.2 Five months after a stem cell transplant for acute myeloid leukaemia in second remission a 45-year-old man is admitted to hospital with fever, anaemia, recent-onset thrombocytopenia and renal impairment. Coagulation screen is normal, haptoglobins are reduced and red cell fragments are seen in the blood film. LDH is 1242 U/l. White cell count and differential are normal. Which of the following is the most appropriate treatment?

☐ **A** Parenteral broad-spectrum antibiotics

☐ **B** Re-induction chemotherapy for relapsed acute myeloid leukaemia

☐ **C** Plasma exchange for fresh-frozen plasma

☐ **D** Daily cryoprecipitate infusion

☐ **E** High-dose steroids

2.3 A 23-year-old woman of Turkish extraction has a 5-year history of systemic lupus erythematosus. She is currently taking prednisolone 7.5 mg daily, which is controlling her arthritic symptoms. She complains of easy tiring in her work as a waitress, which prompts blood tests. These show: white blood cell (WBC) 3.2, haemoglobin (Hb) 8.6, haematocrit (Hct) 0.255, mean corpuscular volume (MCV) 105.5, mean corpuscular haemoglobin (MCH) 35.5, red cell distribution width (RDW) 10.5, platelets (Plts) 149, mean platelet volume (MPV) 7.4, reticulocytes 6.3%, ESR 24 mm/h. Which of the following are most likely to be responsible for her anaemia?

☐ **A** Anaemia of chronic disease

☐ **B** Iron deficiency

☐ **C** Autoimmune haemolytic anaemia

☐ **D** Hypothyroidism

☐ **E** Thalassaemia trait

Answers on pages 95–11

2.4 A 56-year-old man is found to have a palpable liver on clinical examination for an insurance medical. Physical examination is otherwise normal. Abdominal ultrasound shows mild enlargement of the spleen but no intra-abdominal lymphadenopathy. He regularly drinks 18 units of alcohol a week and had suffered haemolytic disease of the newborn, which required exchange transfusion as a baby, and required 12 units red cell transfusion after a transurethral resection of the prostate (TURP) 2 years ago. Blood count:

WBC × 10⁹/l	RBC × 10¹²/l	Hb g/dl	Hct ratio	MCV Fl	MCH pg	MCHC g/dl	RDW	Plt × 10⁹/l
Blood count								
4–11	M 4.7–6.1; F 4.2–5.4	M 13–17.5; F 12–16	M 0.42–0.50; F 0.37–0.47	80–99	27–31	32–35	11.5–14.5	150–400
Blood cultures								
6.9	3.19	9.6	0.313	98	30.1	30.6	17.0	14

Manual differential: neutrophils 75%, lymphocytes 17%, monocytes 4%, eosinophils 1%, myelocytes 1%, metamyelocytes 2%, nucleated red blood cells 2/100 WBC. ESR 15 mm/h. Coagulation screen: normal. Liver biopsy is performed and this is reported as showing myeloid precursors and erythroblast in the liver parenchyma. Bone marrow examination is most likely to show:

☐ **A** Acute megakaryoblastic leukaemia

☐ **B** Aplastic anaemia

☐ **C** Dry tap aspirate with increased reticulin on trephine biopsy

☐ **D** Well differentiated adenocarcinoma of prostate

☐ **E** Gaucher disease

2.5 A 23-three year-old woman is seen in the A&E department with a swollen painful left calf. She had previously suffered a deep vein thrombosis (DVT) in the same leg during her only pregnancy, but no precipitating cause could be found on this occasion. There was no other significant personal or family medical history and she had had no operations. Following the local algorithm for DVT diagnosis she is found to have an elevation of D-dimers and is started on low-molecular-weight heparin (LMWH) injections. Doppler ultrasound performed 2 days later confirms a DVT and she is commenced on warfarin and After 2 weeks attending the hospital anticoagulant clinic she requests transfer of her anticoagulant control to her local GP's surgery, which is geographically more convenient. At her first attendance there the following investigations were performed:

- prothrombin time (PT) 28 (11–14 s)
- International Normalised Ratio (INR) 2.9
- activated partial thromboplastin time (APTT) 38 (25–35 s)
- thrombin time (TT) 16 (5–20 s)
- protein C 0.45 (0.70–1.4)
- protein S 0.65 (0.70–1.4)
- antithrombin 0.95 (.50–1.5)
- screen for factor V Leiden by polymerase chain reaction (PCR) negative
- screen for prothrombin gene mutation by PCR: negative.

Which one of the following is the most appropriate action:

- ☐ **A** Perform activated protein C resistance testing
- ☐ **B** Advise life-long warfarin anticoagulation
- ☐ **C** Screen close family members for protein C deficiency
- ☐ **D** Increase the dose of warfarin
- ☐ **E** Continue warfarin at same dose

Answers on pages 95–11

2.6   Following the diagnosis of nodular sclerosing Hodgkin's disease by biopsy of cervical lymph node a 24-year-old man receives ABVD (adriamycin, bleomycin, vinblastine and dacarbazine) chemotherapy, but after three courses he attends the A&E department complaining of weakness and is found to have a haemoglobin level of 4 g/dl. The hospital computed pathology system showed that a week before his haemoglobin was 6 g/dl and that he was blood group A Rh positive, cytomegalovirus (CMV) antibody positive. Blood pressure is 135/85 mmHg, pulse 90 reg. Which of the following transfusion options is most appropriate?

    ☐   **A**   Irradiated fully crossmatched red cells

    ☐   **B**   Non-irradiated grouped but not matched

    ☐   **C**   Non-irradiated CMV-negative fully matched red cells

    ☐   **D**   Washed irradiated fully matched red cells

    ☐   **E**   Fresh whole blood

2.7   A 78-year-old man presents with symptoms of anaemia. One examination he has five finger-breadth firm splenomegaly and a liver that is just palpable. Blood count shows white blood cell (WBC) 3.8×10^9/l, haemoglobin (Hb) 9.1 g/dl, mean corpuscular volume (MCV) 90 fl, platelets 103×10^9/l, differential neutrophils 80%, lymphocytes 11%, monocytes 3%, metamyelocytes 3%, basophils 3%, nucleated red blood cells 2/100 WBC. Urea and electrolytes are normal. Bone marrow aspirate produced a dry tap and trephine biopsy showed increased reticulin. Which of the following variations in red cell shape (poikilocytosis) would you expect to find on the blood film?

    ☐   **A**   Burr cells

    ☐   **B**   Helmet cells

    ☐   **C**   Tear drops

    ☐   **D**   Elliptocytes

    ☐   **E**   Pencil cells

2.8   **Which one of the following disorders is found more frequently in African countries rather than countries bordering the Mediterranean?**

☐ **A** Beta-thalassaemia trait

☐ **B** Glucose-6-phosphate dehydrogenase (G6PD) deficiency

☐ **C** Leishmaniasis

☐ **D** Pernicious anaemia

☐ **E** Sickle cell disease

2.9   **Which one of the following thrombocytopenic conditions is usually associated with abnormal coagulation screening test results?**

☐ **A** Idiopathic thrombocytopenic purpura

☐ **B** Thrombotic thrombocytopenic purpura

☐ **C** Haemolytic–uraemic syndrome

☐ **D** Disseminated intravascular coagulation

☐ **E** May–Hegglin anomaly

2.10   **A 70-year-old woman is admitted with a fractured femur. Bones showed a generalised osteopenia on X-ray. Protein electrophoresis showed an IgG kappa paraprotein at a concentration of 8 g/l. Urine shows no Bence-Jones protein. Creatinine was elevated to 140 mmol/l with a urea of 14 mmol/l. Which one of the following is in favour of a diagnosis of plasma cell myeloma rather than monoclonal gammopathy of undetermined significance (MGUS):**

☐ **A** Diffuse increase in gamma globulin level

☐ **B** Plasma cell marrow infiltration of 5%

☐ **C** Normal serum calcium

☐ **D** Patchy PET-FDG active lesions in lumbar and thoracic vertebrae

☐ **E** No increase in level of paraprotein over six months' observation

Answers on pages 95–11?

2.11 A 64-year-old man is admitted to hospital with a week's history of increasing confusion, nosebleeds, shortness of breath on exertion and peripheral oedema. He has been taking bendrofluazide for a number of years for essential hypertension. On examination he is pale and afebrile. There is a generalised lymphadenopathy and the spleen is just palpable below the left costal margin. Blood count shows white blood cell (WBC) 34.3×10^9/l, haemoglobin (Hb) 9.2 g/dl, platelets 120×10^9/l. Differential: neutrophils 10%, lymphocytes 85%, monocytes 5%; erythrocyte sedimentation rate (ESR) 140 mm/h; C-reactive protein (CRP) 10 µg/l. Renal function shows a urea of 15 mmol/l and creatinine of 200 mmol/l. Which one of the following tests is the most useful to explain his confusion?

☐ **A** Electrolyte measurement

☐ **B** Plasma viscosity

☐ **C** Blood cultures

☐ **D** Screen for drugs of addiction

☐ **E** Plasma bicarbonate

2.12 Which of the following provide the earliest indicator of intravascular haemolysis?

☐ **A** Urinary haemosiderin

☐ **B** Elevated reticulocyte count

☐ **C** Elevated conjugated hyperbilirubin

☐ **D** Reduced plasma haptoglobin

☐ **E** Marrow erythroid hyperplasia

2.13 A 25-year-old woman seen in the Dermatology Out-Patient Department for the treatment of dermatitis herpetiformis is noted to be peripherally and centrally cyanosed. Physical examination of chest and cardiovascular system is normal. Oxygen saturation as measured by pulse oximetry is normal. Which of the following is the most appropriate investigation?

☐ **A** Cardiac catheterisation

☐ **B** Arterial blood gas measurement

☐ **C** G6PD measurement

☐ **D** Cardiac ECHO

☐ **E** Spectroscopic examination of haemoglobin

2.14 A 67-year-old man is admitted with a history of two days' headache and confusion. He has been taking warfarin for atrial fibrillation for the last two years. Urgent computed tomography (CT) scan of the head demonstrates a sub-dural haematoma with mid-line shift. Coagulation screen shows: APTT 50 s (25–35 s), prothrombin time 40 s (11–14 s), INR 7.0 (1.0–1.3), fibrinogen 3.2 (2–5 g/l), D-dimers 0.6 (0–0.4 µg/ml). Which one of the following statements is most likely to be correct?

- [ ] **A** Sudden reduction in his regular alcohol intake has caused warfarin over-anticoagulation
- [ ] **B** The coagulation abnormalities are most likely to be secondary to disseminated intravascular coagulation (DIC) rather than warfarin overdose
- [ ] **C** Increase in spinach consumption from his allotment has caused warfarin over-anticoagulation
- [ ] **D** Congenital coagulopathy should be seriously considered as a cause of his abnormal coagulation
- [ ] **E** Prescription of simvastatin 2 weeks ago has caused warfarin over-anticoagulation

2.15 A 23-year-old woman presents with right-sided abdominal pain, ascites and hepatosplenomegaly with tenderness over the liver. Abdominal Doppler ultrasound examination shows no flow in the hepatic veins. The following haematological investigations are performed: WBC 15.5×10^9/l, haemoglobin 12.5 g/dl, mean corpuscular volume (MCV) 70 fl, MCH 24 pg, platelets 835×10^9/l, coagulation screen normal, protein C 80 U/dl (normal range 70–140), protein S 90 U/dl (normal range 60–140), antithrombin 110 U/dl (normal range 80–120), activated protein c (APC) resistance 2.38 (normal range 2.18–2.52), ferritin 10 µg. l (normal 15–2000). Her contraceptive pill is stopped. Anticoagulation with heparin/warfarin and oral iron is started. After one month her blood count shows: white blood cell (WBC) 14.5×10^9/l, haemoglobin 17.5 g/dl, mean corpuscular volume (MCV) 72 fl, platelets 721×10^9/l. Which of the following is the most likely haematological diagnosis?

- [ ] **A** Chronic myeloid leukaemia
- [ ] **B** Factor V Leiden heterozygote
- [ ] **C** Iron deficiency anaemia
- [ ] **D** Primary polycythaemia rubra vera
- [ ] **E** Primary thrombocythaemia

Answers on pages 95–11.

2.16 **Which one of the following is true of fresh-frozen plasma (FFP)?**

☐ **A** It is the optimal replacement fluid following major burns

☐ **B** Group O FFP may be given to recipients of any ABO group

☐ **C** It is approved for the urgent correction of over-anticoagulation with heparin

☐ **D** It contains all the coagulation factors, albumin and immunoglobulin

☐ **E** It takes 5–10 minutes to thaw before administration

2.17 **A 68-year-old woman visits her GP complaining of chilblains. She is noted to have peripheral cyanosis without other abnormalities of physical examination and some screening investigations, including a blood count, are performed. This screen shows white blood cells (WBC) 8.5 × 10⁹/l, (differential: neutrophils 82%, lymphocytes 15%, monocytes 3%), platelets 148 × 10⁹/l. Film comment is 'heavy cold agglutinates present, sample processed at 37 °C'. Which one of the following is the most likely cause of her haematological abnormalities?**

☐ **A** B-cell chronic lymphocytic leukaemia

☐ **B** Glandular fever

☐ **C** Idiopathic cold haemagglutinin disease

☐ **D** *Mycoplasma* chest infection

☐ **E** Tertiary syphilis

2.18 You are asked to see a 21-year-old man on the ENT ward who has had excessive bleeding after tonsillectomy, necessitating return to theatre on two occasions. He has not had any history of other surgery. His mother has a history of menorrhagia and a maternal aunt bled excessively following tonsillectomy in childhood. Results show white blood cell (WBC) 8.5×10^9/l, haemoglobin 12.5 g/dl, platelets 150×10^9/l, prothrombin time 15 s (normal range 12–17), APTT 39 s (normal range 24–38), thrombin time 17 s (normal range 14–22), fibrinogen 3.8 g/l (normal range 2–5), platelet function analyser PFA-100 closure times with collagen/adrenaline 210 s, (normal less than 116) with collagen/ADP 190 s (normal less than 116 s). Which one of the following is the most likely diagnosis?

☐ **A** Aspirin effect

☐ **B** Haemophilia A

☐ **C** Heparin sample contamination

☐ **D** Poor surgical haemostasis

☐ **E** Von Willebrand disease

2.19 A 24-year-old man has noted for the last 2 months that his face is swollen in the mornings. He has lost 10 kg in weight over the last 6 months and has an intermittent fever. He is a non-smoker, and drinks alcohol very rarely. On examination his external jugular veins are dilated. His chest X-ray shows a mediastinal mass. Which of the following is the most likely cause of his superior vena caval obstruction?

☐ **A** Adenocarcinoma of lung

☐ **B** Hodgkin's disease

☐ **C** Sarcoidosis

☐ **D** Seminoma

☐ **E** Tuberculosis

Answers on pages 95–11?

2.20 An 80-year-old woman presents with a transient ischaemic attack with a 5 minute loss of power in her right side. She has no previous history of note, has been very well and is taking no medicines. On examination, the day after the attack, there were no residual neurological signs and examination of her cardiovascular system is normal. On investigation her white blood cell (WBC) is 11.5×10^9/l, haemoglobin 12.5 g/dl, mean corpuscular volume (MCV) 94 fl, MCH 29 pg, platelets 1135×10^9/l, erythrocyte sedimentation rate (ESR) 2 mm in first hour, ferritin 23 µg/l (normal range 15–200). Which one of the following is the most appropriate treatment?

☐ **A** Warfarin anticoagulation

☐ **B** Heparin anticoagulation

☐ **C** Oral iron

☐ **D** Vincristine

☐ **E** Hydroxycarbamide

2.21 A 14-year-old girl presents with symptoms of anaemia, nosebleeds and purpura of her feet. On examination there is no enlargement of liver, spleen or lymph nodes. A blood count shows white blood cell (WBC) 2.3×10^9/l, haemoglobin 6.0 g/dl, platelets 9×10^9/l. Bone marrow aspirate is hypercellular, showing 95% blasts, a few of which contain Auer rods. Cytogenetic analysis shows translocation between chromosomes 9 and 21. Which one of the following statements about her treatment is true?

☐ **A** If a matched unrelated donor was found, then bone marrow transplant in first remission would be her best treatment option

☐ **B** Induction chemotherapy contains high-dose steroids and vincristine

☐ **C** The morphology and cytogenetics are compatible with acute promyelocytic leukaemia

☐ **D** This cytogenetic abnormality is associated with Philadelphia chromosome

☐ **E** Induction chemotherapy would usually consist of cytosine and an anthracycline

2.22 A 35-year-old woman is admitted to the Emergency Department at 8 am after having an epileptic fit on the station platform. A St John's Ambulance volunteer witnesses this. On examination, she is confused, has been incontinent of urine and has a temperature of 37.5 °C. Her husband is contacted at work who states that she has been suffering from a diarrhoeal illness for the last few days and had gone to bed with a headache the previous evening. She has no previous history of epilepsy and is taking no medications regularly. Blood count shows white blood cell (WBC) 12.6×10^9/l, haemoglobin 8.6 g/dl, platelets 23×10^9/l. Blood film examination confirms thrombocytopenia and shows occasional fragmented cells. Reticulocyte count is 4.6%. Biochemical tests show normal electrolytes, a creatinine of 146 µmol/l and urea of 8.8 mmol/l. Liver function tests are normal except a bilirubin of 29 µmol/l and LDH 1300 U/l. Which one of the following statements is least likely to be true?

☐ **A** The clinical and pathological features may all be related to the post-ictal state

☐ **B** Increased levels of high molecular weight von Willebrand's factor may be found in her blood

☐ **C** Enteric infection with *Escherichia coli* may be causally related to her illness

☐ **D** The elevated LDH is likely to be of red cell origin

☐ **E** Coagulation screening tests in this disorder are usually normal

2.23 An 18-year-old woman complains of tiredness. She is a vegetarian and her periods last 6 days of a 28-day cycle. There is no significant previous medical history, and no abnormal features on examination. Blood count shows white blood cell (WBC) 4.1×10^9/l, haemoglobin 10.1 g/dl, mean corpuscular volume (MCV) 63 fl, platelets 492×10^9/l. Which one of the following is not in keeping with her clinical and pathological features?

☐ **A** Low serum ferritin

☐ **B** Stainable bone marrow iron

☐ **C** Low transferrin saturation

☐ **D** High erythrocyte zinc protoporphyrin

☐ **E** Normal haemoglobin A_2 level

2.24 A 5-year-old boy of Turkish extraction is referred to the school's medical service because of developmental delay. He is noted to be pale and has a palpable spleen. Blood count shows white blood cell (WBC) 5.5×10^9/l, haemoglobin 4.3 g/dl, mean corpuscular volume (MCV) 62 fl, platelets 323×10^9/l. Which one of the following is not in keeping with a diagnosis of β-thalassaemia major?

☐ **A** Haemoglobin F level of 90%

☐ **B** Nucleated red cells in the peripheral blood

☐ **C** Normal serum ferritin

☐ **D** Prognathism

☐ **E** Diastolic murmur at the cardiac apex

2.25 A 55-year-old woman on the Intensive Care Unit following a road traffic accident has routine haematology investigations performed. These show WBC 12.3×10^9/l, haemoglobin 11.4 g/dl, platelets 304×10^9/l. Prothrombin time 14 s (control 13 s), APTT 41 s (control 38 s), thrombin time 30 s, (control 12 s). Which one of the following should be done?

☐ **A** Administration of 2 units of fresh-frozen plasma

☐ **B** Transfusion of 10 units of cryoprecipitate

☐ **C** Repeat coagulation screen on fresh sample

☐ **D** Measurement of fibrin degradation products (FDPs)

☐ **E** Administration of vitamin K

2.26 A 30-year-old woman develops pleuritic left-sided chest pain one week after normal vaginal delivery of a six-pound baby boy. On examination she is noted to have a swollen left leg and Doppler ultrasound confirms the presence of thrombus in the deep venous system. There is no personal or family history of thrombosis. Which one of the following investigations is most appropriate?

☐ **A** Measurement of plasma antithrombin

☐ **B** Coagulation screen

☐ **C** Screening for factor V Leiden mutation by APC resistance

☐ **D** Protein S measurement

☐ **E** Measurement of coagulation factor IX

2.27 The patient above commenced conventional heparin by intravenous infusion at a rate of 1000 units per hour. Six hours after starting the infusion her coagulation tests shows: INR 1.2, APTT 68 s (control 38 s). Which one of the following actions is most appropriate?

☐ **A** Stop intravenous heparin and give 30 mg oral warfarin

☐ **B** Convert to therapeutic dose of once-daily subcutaneous low molecular weight heparin

☐ **C** Increase heparin infusion rate to 1500 units per hour

☐ **D** Continue heparin infusion at current rate

☐ **E** Stop all anticoagulant treatment

2.28 A 55-year-old man attends his doctor's surgery complaining of a lump beneath his left jaw. On examination he is found to have a mild generalised lymphadenopathy. His blood count shows white blood cell (WBC) 50.5×10^9/l, haemoglobin 12.6 g/dl, platelets 183×10^9/l. Which one of the following would be most against the diagnosis of chronic lymphocytic leukaemia?

☐ **A** Peripheral blood lymphocytes expressing both CD5 and CD19 antigens

☐ **B** Reduced levels of IgG and IgA immunoglobulins

☐ **C** Positive direct antiglobulin test

☐ **D** Presence of smear cells on peripheral blood film

☐ **E** Balanced expression of kappa and lambda light chain of surface immunoglobulin on blood lymphocytes

2.29 A 14-year-old girl with Down's syndrome and epilepsy has a screening full blood count performed after an increase in the incidence of her fits. This shows white blood cell (WBC) 4.3×10^9/l, haemoglobin 11.0 g/dl, mean corpuscular volume (MCV) 103 fl, platelets 165×10^9/l. Which one of the following should not be considered as a cause of her macrocytosis?

☐ **A** Antiepileptic drugs

☐ **B** Subacute hepatitis

☐ **C** Folic acid deficiency

☐ **D** Multiple myeloma

☐ **E** Autoimmune haemolytic anaemia

Answers on pages 95–112

2.30 The mother of a 12-year-old boy with classic haemophilia requests a consultation because of a persistent haemarthrosis of his right ankle. This joint frequently gives him a problem. He is on a regimen of prophylactic alternate-day factor VIII, given by his mother. On examination he has a hot, tender, swollen left ankle. He is otherwise well and there are no other abnormal features on examination. Which one of the following is the most relevant investigation to perform?

- ☐ **A** Blood count
- ☐ **B** Factor IX level
- ☐ **C** Factor VIII inhibitor screen
- ☐ **D** Urate level
- ☐ **E** Joint aspiration

2.31 A 30-year-old woman is admitted with a deep venous thrombosis. A blood count demonstrates a pancytopenia with a haemoglobin of 5 g/dl and she receives a 4-unit red cell transfusion. Following this she is noted to have dark urine and no red cells are seen in the urine on microscopy. Direct antiglobulin test is negative and repeat blood grouping confirms her ABO type and no atypical red cell antibodies are discovered. Which one of the following investigations is now most appropriate?

- ☐ **A** Donath–Landsteiner test
- ☐ **B** MSU for MC & S
- ☐ **C** Ham's acid serum haemolysis test
- ☐ **D** Urinary haemosiderin
- ☐ **E** Measurement of CD55 and CD59 surface antigen on peripheral blood leucocytes and platelets

2.32 Which one of the following statements about cryoprecipitate is incorrect?

- ☐ **A** It is prepared by thawing fresh-frozen plasma
- ☐ **B** It is rich in fibrinogen
- ☐ **C** It is free of risk of hepatitis transmission
- ☐ **D** It may correct the platelet defect found in uraemic patients
- ☐ **E** It contains factor VIII and von Willebrand's factor

2.33   A 60-year-old woman with high-grade B cell lymphoma receives treatment with CHOP chemotherapy. Ten days after completion of her first course she is admitted to hospital with bilateral bronchopneumonia, requiring treatment with ventilation in the Intensive Care Unit. Her blood count shows white blood cell (WBC) $0.9 \times 10^9/l$ (neutrophils 0), haemoglobin 10.1 g/dl, platelets $106 \times 10^9/l$. Which one of the following statements concerning her treatment with granulocyte colony-stimulating factor (G-CSF) is true?

☐   **A**   Prophylactic G-CSF administration to ameliorate neutropenia during future chemotherapy should be administered before and during the course of chemotherapy

☐   **B**   Bone pain is a side-effect of treatment that resolves shortly before granulocyte recovery

☐   **C**   Extending the time between courses of chemotherapy to allow haematopoietic recovery is preferable to cytokine stimulation of granulocyte recovery

☐   **D**   G-CSF carries no risk of viral transmission

☐   **E**   G-CSF stimulates haematopoietic stem cells into granulocyte differentiation

2.34   A 20-year-old woman being investigated for anaemia has the following blood count: white blood cell (WBC) $1.6 \times 10^9/l$ (neutrophils 0.6), haemoglobin 7.0 g/dl, MCV 102 fl, platelets $23 \times 10^9/l$. Bone marrow aspirate and trephine biopsy are hypocellular, showing residual lymphocytes and scattered eosinophils only. Which one of the following features in her history is not relevant to her diagnosis?

☐   **A**   Recovery from hepatitis A infection 3 months previously

☐   **B**   Recent febrile illness associated with high titres against parvovirus B19

☐   **C**   Positive Ham's acid serum haemolysis test

☐   **D**   Estranged husband is on busulfan treatment for chronic myeloid leukaemia

☐   **E**   Phenylbutazone treatment for ankylosing spondylitis

Answers on pages 95–112

2.35   A patient with a first pulmonary embolus has been on continuous intravenous heparin for 5 days and has received one dose of 10 mg warfarin 12 hours before blood is drawn for coagulation tests: these show an activated partial thromboplastin time (APTT) ratio of 1.7, and an international normalised ratio (INR) of 1.8. Which one of the following is incorrect?

- ☐ **A**   The heparin should be increased
- ☐ **B**   The INR result shows the effect of over-heparinisation
- ☐ **C**   The patient is unusually sensitive to the effect of warfarin
- ☐ **D**   The aimed-for INR range in this patient is 3–4.5
- ☐ **E**   The INR is the patient's prothrombin time in seconds divided by the normal control time in seconds

2.36   A 60-year-old Asian woman has a haemoglobin of 6.6 g/dl (MCV 63 fl). Which one of the following is least likely to be causally related to her anaemia?

- ☐ **A**   History of pernicious anaemia treated with quarterly B12 injections
- ☐ **B**   Regular ibuprofen ingestion for osteoarthritis
- ☐ **C**   Vegan diet
- ☐ **D**   Beta-thalassaemia trait
- ☐ **E**   Elevated thyroid-stimulating hormone (TSH) and low free thyroxine

2.37   In a patient with chronic renal failure on replacement erythropoietin (EPO) injections, which one of the following is not a recognised unwanted effect of this treatment?

- ☐ **A**   Hypertension
- ☐ **B**   Increased risk of thrombosis
- ☐ **C**   Pure red cell aplasia
- ☐ **D**   Anorexia and malaise
- ☐ **E**   Local pain at injection site

2.38 A 54-year old man has: white blood cell (WBC) 5.4×10^9/l, haemoglobin 10.4 g/dl, platelets 135×10^9/l. Differential white cell count shows neutrophils 87%, lymphocytes 6%, monocytes 3%, metamyelocytes 3%, promyelocytes 1%, and nucleated red cells 3 per 100 white cells. Which one of the following is not an appropriate investigation to elucidate the cause of the abnormal blood picture?

☐ **A** Chest X-ray

☐ **B** Haemoglobin electrophoresis

☐ **C** Bone marrow aspirate

☐ **D** Prostate specific antigen (PSA)

☐ E Abdominal ultrasound

2.39 Which one of the following statements regarding human blood groups is true?

☐ **A** Naturally occurring anti-A and anti-B antibodies can be both IgG and IgM

☐ **B** A minority of people secrete their ABO antigen in saliva and other body fluids

☐ **C** The ABO type of individuals can change during some illnesses, eg acute myeloid leukaemia

☐ **D** Group A is the commonest blood group in all races

☐ **E** People of blood group O are universal donors for fresh-frozen plasma

2.40 Eight days after commencing intravenous conventional heparin therapy for a deep venous thrombosis a patient's routine full blood count shows a platelet count of 19×10^9/l. This is confirmed on a fresh sample and the records show a normal platelet count on admission to hospital a week before. Which one of the following actions is most appropriate?

☐ **A** Stop heparin and commence heparinoid

☐ **B** Change conventional heparin to low molecular weight heparin

☐ **C** Stop heparin and commence warfarin

☐ **D** Stop all anticoagulant therapy until the results of anti-PF4–heparin complex ELISA are available

☐ **E** Stop all anticoagulants and transfuse platelet concentrate

Answers on pages 95–112

2.41 A 30-year-old man, previously well, presents to the Emergency Department with a grand mal fit. On examination his temperature is 37.8 °C and he is post-ictal. He has a petechial rash on his lower limbs. His laboratory investigations are as follows: haemoglobin 12.5 g/dl, white cell count (WBC) 10.0 × 10⁹/l with a normal differential, platelets 20 × 10⁹/l, reticulocytes 205 × 10⁹/l (normal range 50–100), PT 14 s (normal range 12–17), APPT 35 s (normal range 24–38) TT 14 s (normal range 14–22), fibrinogen 4.5 g/l (normal range 2–5), D-dimer 0 mg/ml, urea 20 mmol/l, sodium 142 mmol/l, potassium 4.1 mmol/l, creatinine 234 mmol/l, aspartate aminotransferase (AST) 23 U/l, alanine aminotransferase (ALT) 40 U/l, alkaline phosphatase (ALP) 95 U/l, bilirubin 40 µmol/l, LDH 950 U/l. Which one of the following is the most likely diagnosis?

☐ **A** Acute glomerulonephritis

☐ **B** Immune thrombocytopenic purpura

☐ C Meningococcal meningitis

☐ **D** Systemic lupus erythematosus

☐ **E** Thrombotic thrombocytopenic purpura

2.42 Mr Smith is undergoing a hip replacement. During surgery, he loses approximately 1 litre of blood and transfusion of 2 units of packed cells is commenced towards the end of the operation. The anaesthetist notices that his pulse has risen to 130 bpm and his blood pressure has fallen to 80/40 mmHg. He is noted to have frank haematuria. Which one of the following is the most likely cause of the sudden deterioration?

☐ **A** Major ABO incompatibility

☐ **B** Myocardial infarction

☐ **C** Overwhelming sepsis

☐ **D** Reaction to anaesthetic drug

☐ **E** Undetected blood loss

Questions: Haematology

2.43 A 20-year-old thin woman presents with right-sided abdominal pain. In her family history her mother had a splenectomy for anaemia and her maternal grandmother had gallstones. On examination she is mildly jaundiced, tender in her right hypochondrium and has 1 cm of splenomegaly. Ultrasound shows gallstones and an enlarged spleen. Investigations show: haemoglobin 10.5 g/dl, mean corpuscular volume (MCV) 102 fl, MCH 31 pg, MCHC 35 g/dl, WBC 10.0×10^9/l with a normal differential, platelets 425×10^9/l, reticulocytes 216×10^9/l (normal range 50–100), urea 5.0 mmol/l, sodium 139 mmol/l , potassium 4.0 mmol/l, creatinine 65 mmol/l, aspartate aminotransferase (AST) 25 U/l, alanine aminotransferase (ALT) 41 U/l, ALP 90 U/l, bilirubin 35 μmol/l, LDH 850 U/l. Which one of the following is the most likely diagnosis?

- **A** Autoimmune haemolytic anaemia
- **B** Chronic myeloid leukaemia
- **C** Hepatitis B
- **D** Hereditary spherocytosis
- **E** Systemic lupus erythematosus

2.44 A 25-year-old student about to sit his final undergraduate examinations notices that his vision has deteriorated markedly in his right eye. On presentation at the Emergency Department he is noted to be a pale, but fit-looking young man. On examination he is found to have 3 cm of splenomegaly and fundal haemorrhages in both eyes, affecting the macula on the right side. A blood count shows haemoglobin 5.5 g/dl, white cell count (WBC) 195×10^9/l (blasts 5%, promyelocytes 10%, myelocytes 34%, metamyelocytes 15%, neutrophils 33%, eosinophils 2%, basophils 1%), platelets 625×10^9/l. Which one of the following is the most likely diagnosis?

- **A** Acute myeloid leukaemia
- **B** Chronic myeloid leukaemia
- **C** Leukaemoid reaction
- **D** Myelofibrosis
- **E** Primary thrombocythaemia

2.45 A 65-year-old woman has a 6-month history of low back pain. She presents to the Emergency Department with weakness in her legs for four days and failure to pass any urine for 24 hours. On examination she is pale and tender over her lumbar spine. Power is grade 4 in both legs with absent reflexes and down-going plantars. Her bladder is palpable to her umbilicus. Her haemoglobin is 10.5 g/dl, mean corpuscular volume (MCV) 102 fl, white cell count (WBC) 3.0×10^9/l with a normal differential, platelets 120×10^9/l, urea 20 mmol/l, sodium 143 mmol/l, potassium 4.9 mmol/l, creatinine 300 mmol/l, AST 15 U/l, ALT 22 U/l, ALP 90 U/l, bilirubin 35 μmol/l, total protein 90 g/l, albumin 25 g/l. X-ray of her lumbar spine shows generalised osteopenia and a lytic lesion is noted in her pelvis. Which one of the following is the most likely diagnosis?

☐ **A** Guillain–Barré syndrome

☐ **B** Metastatic breast carcinoma

☐ **C** Multiple myeloma

☐ **D** Non-Hodgkin's lymphoma

☐ **E** Thrombotic thrombocytopenic purpura

2.46 A 70-year-old woman is noted by her family to be pale and slightly confused. On examination she is anaemic and slightly jaundiced. Pulse is 80 bpm, JVP not raised with a negative hepatojugular reflux and two heart sounds, with no added sounds. Her respiratory system is normal. Haemoglobin 3.5 g/dl, mean corpuscular volume (MCV) 120 fl, MCH 34 pg, MCHC 35 g/dl, WBC 3.0×10^9/l, platelets 105×10^9/l, urea 5.0 mmol/l, sodium 141 mmol/l, potassium 4.5 mmol/l, creatinine 65 μmol/l, aspartate aminotransferase (AST) 35 U/l, alanine aminotransferase (ALT) 32 U/l, ALP 50 U/l, bilirubin 35 μmol/l, LDH 850 U/l. Which one of the following would be the most appropriate management of this condition?

☐ **A** Vitamin B_{12}, folic acid and iron supplements

☐ **B** Vitamin B_{12}, folic acid and iron supplements and slow transfusion of 1–2 units of packed cells if clinically indicated

☐ **C** Intravenous folinic acid

☐ **D** Immediate transfusion of 4 units of packed cells

☐ **E** Transfusion of 4 units of fresh-frozen plasma

2.47   A 20-year-old man of Greek origin presents with a three-day history of pallor and dark urine. He was about to go to Kenya on holiday. In his family history a brother had a similar episode some years ago following a course of Septrin. On examination, apart from pallor, there is nothing to find. Results show: haemoglobin 5.5 g/dl, mean corpuscular volume (MCV) 105 fl, MCH 27 pg, MCHC 36 g/dl, white cell count (WBC) 8.5×10^9/l with a normal differential, platelets 425×10^9/l, reticulocytes 196×10^9/l (normal range 50–100), urea 3.5 mmol/l, sodium 138 mmol/l, potassium 4.0 mmol/l, creatinine 70 μmol/l, aspartate aminotransferase (AST) 31 U/l, alanine aminotransferase (ALT) 27 U/l, ALP 100 U/l, bilirubin 75 μmol/l, LDH 1250 U/l. His blood film shows blister cells. Which one of the following is the most likely diagnosis?

☐ **A**   Aplastic anaemia

☐ **B**   Autoimmune haemolytic anaemia

☐ **C**   Glucose-6-phosphate dehydrogenase (G6PD) deficiency

☐ **D**   Hepatitis B

☐ **E**   Hereditary spherocytosis

2.48   A 70-year-old man presents with a history of tiredness and increasing shortness of breath. On examination he is clinically anaemic. On investigation his haemoglobin is 8.5 g/dl, mean corpuscular volume (MCV) 110 fl, MCH 24 pg, MCHC 29 g/dl, white cell count (WBC) 10.4×10^9/l, platelets 80×10^9/l, normal urea and electrolytes and liver function tests, serum iron 45 μmol/l (normal range 14–29), total iron-binding capacity (TIBC) 64 μmol/l (normal range 45–72), ferritin 453 μg/l (normal range 15–200). Bone marrow aspirate shows abnormal erythropoiesis and increased iron in the stores and erythroid series. Which one of the following is the most likely diagnosis?

☐ **A**   Acute myeloid leukaemia

☐ **B**   Haemochromatosis

☐ **C**   Multiple myeloma

☐ **D**   Myelodysplastic syndrome

☐ **E**   Sideroblastic anaemia

Answers on pages 95–11?

2.49   A 20-year-old African refugee presents with sudden onset of a dense right sided hemiparesis. He speaks little English but from friends it appears that he has no previous medical history of note but two siblings died in infancy. On examination he has a right hemiparesis and 3 cm splenomegaly. On investigation his haemoglobin is 8.5 g/dl, mean corpuscular volume (MCV) 102 fl, MCH 33 pg, MCHC 32.5 g/dl, white cell count (WBC) 12.5×10^9/l with a neutrophil leucocytosis, platelets 120×10^9/l, reticulocytes 221×10^9/l (normal range 50–100), urea 3.5 mmol/l, sodium 140 mmol/l, potassium 4.0 mmol/l, creatinine 70 μmol/l, aspartate aminotransferase (AST) 30 U/l, alanine aminotransferase (ALT) 62 U/l, ALP 52 U/l, bilirubin 55 μmol/l, LDH 1128 U/l. His blood film shows numerous sickled cells. Which one of the following is the most important immediate management of his condition?

☐ **A** Immediate exchange transfusion

☐ **B** Intravenous antibiotics

☐ **C** Pain relief

☐ **D** Rehydration

☐ **E** Top-up transfusion

2.50   You are called to see a 28-year-old Hong Kong Chinese lady who is 28 weeks' pregnant (first pregnancy). She has no previous history of note. She is now pre-eclamptic and the fetus has been noted on ultrasound to be hydropic. Results show: haemoglobin 10.5 g/dl, mean corpuscular volume (MCV) 65 fl, MCH 22 pg, MCHC 37 g/dl, white cell count (WBC) 11.5×10^9/l, platelets 120×10^9/l, prothrombin time 12 s (normal range 12–17), APPT 29 s (normal range 24–38), thrombin time 16 s (normal range 14–22), fibrinogen 3.2 g/l (normal range 2–5), urea 9.5 mmol/l, sodium 137 mmol/l, potassium 4.0 mmol/l, creatinine 110 μmol/l, aspartate aminotransferase (AST) 53 U/l, alanine aminotransferase (ALT) 52 U/l, ALP 110 U/l, bilirubin 36 μmol/l, LDH 700 U/l. Which one of following is the most likely cause of the hydropic fetus?

☐ **A** HELLP syndrome

☐ **B** Hepatitis C

☐ **C** Pre-eclampsia

☐ **D** Septicaemia

☐ **E** Beta-thalassaemia major

JET LIBRARY

Respiratory Medicine

Best of Five

Questions

RESPIRATORY MEDICINE 'BEST OF FIVE' QUESTIONS

For each of the questions select the ONE most appropriate answer from the options provided.

3.1 **A 35-year-old White woman comes to see you concerned about her new diagnosis of sarcoidosis. Which one of the following would be a bad prognostic factor?**

☐ **A** Current smoking history

☐ **B** Erythema nodosum

☐ **C** Being White

☐ **D** Lupus pernio

☐ **E** High serum ACE level

3.2 **A 54-year-old old heavy smoker with severe chronic obstructive pulmonary disease (COPD) has been diagnosed as having non-small-cell carcinoma. Surgical resection would require a pneumonectomy. Which of the following is a contraindication for proposed radical (ie potentially curative) surgery?**

☐ **A** Hypercalcaemia

☐ **B** Pleural effusion

☐ **C** Mediastinal lymph nodes 0.8 cm

☐ **D** Clubbing

☐ **E** Forced expiratory volume in one second (FEV_1) of 1.6

3.3 **Which one of the following has been shown epidemiologically to increase your chances of developing asthma?**

☐ **A** Living in the countryside

☐ **B** Having TB as a child

☐ **C** Living in a developing country

☐ **D** Being the youngest sibling within a large family

☐ **E** Being the oldest sibling within a large family

3.4   **A 46-year-old non-smoker develops breathlessness 3 months after starting a job in a pet shop. Which one of the following would suggest a diagnosis of extrinsic allergic alveolitis?**

☐ **A** Heavy smoking history

☐ **B** Basal fibrosis on chest X-ray

☐ **C** Chest heaviness, fevers but no wheeze in the evenings

☐ **D** High levels of IgE and eosinophilia

☐ **E** History of atopy

3.5   **A 50-year-old quartz miner is diagnosed with chronic silicosis. Which one of the following statements is true about his condition?**

☐ **A** He is at increased risk of tuberculosis

☐ **B** His lung function tests will show restrictive spirometry

☐ **C** His CT scan will show basal fibrosis

☐ **D** His CT scan will show apical fibrosis

☐ **E** He can continue in his job if his lung function is normal

3.6   **Which one of the following statements is true concerning pulmonary haemorrhage?**

☐ **A** Decreased KCO

☐ **B** Decreased TLCO

☐ **C** It improves gas diffusion from alveoli to capillary

☐ **D** It is typically seen with polyarteritis nodosa

☐ **E** Can occur in rheumatoid arthritis

Answers on pages 115–12.

.7   **A 28-year-old patient is referred to you by his GP with a history of pan-sinusitis as a child and frequent chest infections. In passing, he tells you that he and his partner have been unsuccessfully trying for a baby. Which one of the following statements is true?**

☐ **A** Absence of vas deferens would make cystic fibrosis the most likely diagnosis

☐ **B** Absence of dextrocardia would exclude primary ciliary dyskinesia

☐ **C** Absence of ΔF508 excludes cystic fibrosis

☐ **D** Recurrent pseudomonas infection would indicate an immunodeficiency

☐ **E** If severe enough, his condition could warrant a single lung transplant

.8   **A Peruvian Indian living at 4600 metres altitude was found to be acutely breathless. Which one of the following possibilities could explain his symptoms?**

☐ **A** His oxygen dissociation curve is shifted to the right

☐ **B** His $p(O_2)$ is 6.1 kPa

☐ **C** His saturations are 81%

☐ **D** His haemoglobin is 15g/dl

☐ **E** He has increased levels of 2,3-diphosphoglycerate (2,3-DPG)

.9   **Which one of the following is a recognised cause of restrictive spirometry?**

☐ **A** Bronchiectasis

☐ **B** Obliterative bronchiolitis

☐ **C** Simple coal worker's pneumoconiosis

☐ **D** Obesity

☐ **E** Asthma

3.10 **A woman with arteriovenous malformation (AVM) is found to have new onset right sided hemiparesis, fever and decreased conscious level. The most likely diagnosis is:**

- ☐ **A** Cerebral abscess
- ☐ **B** Bacterial meningitis
- ☐ **C** Tuberculous meningitis
- ☐ **D** Ruptured cerebral AVM
- ☐ **E** Thrombo-embolic stroke

3.11 **A 64-year-old woman presents with community-acquired pneumonia (CAP). Which of the following features on admission would indicate a poor prognosis?**

- ☐ **A** White cell count of 18×10^9/l
- ☐ **B** Blood pressure 110/70 mmHg
- ☐ **C** Respiratory rate 35/min
- ☐ **D** Pyrexia of 40 °C
- ☐ **E** Rigors

3.12 **Which one of the following statements is true concerning ventilation (V) and perfusion (Q) in the lung while standing up:**

- ☐ **A** Perfusion is greatest at the apex
- ☐ **B** Ventilation is greatest at the apex
- ☐ **C** V/Q highest at base
- ☐ **D** V/Q highest at apex
- ☐ **E** V/Q matching decreases during exercise

3.13 **Carcinoid lung tumours:**

- ☐ **A** Often cavitate
- ☐ **B** Are usually visible on bronchoscopy
- ☐ **C** Are often associated with flushing and sweating
- ☐ **D** Are associated with smoking
- ☐ **E** Often recur after surgery

Answers on pages 115–12.

.14   Apical fibrosis:

☐ **A** Commonly occurs in ankylosing spondylitis

☐ **B** Can be seen in simple coal worker's pneumoconiosis

☐ **C** Occurs in farmer's lung

☐ **D** Can be detected in byssinosis

☐ **E** Occurs in asbestosis

.15   A young man presents with a spontaneous pneumothorax. Which one of the following statements is correct?

☐ **A** Smoking is not a risk factor in the context of a normal chest X-ray and normal lung function

☐ **B** A smoking history would exclude a diagnosis of Langerhans' cell histiocytosis

☐ **C** If associated with cystic lung lesions, could be due to lymphangioleiomatosis (LAM)

☐ **D** Commonly complicates lung disease in cystic fibrosis

☐ **E** If a complete pneumothorax is detected in someone with normally underlying lung parenchyma, a chest drain should be inserted without attempting aspiration

.16   A 39-year-old woman with asthma has a strongly positive skin-prick test to *Aspergillus fumigatus.* You think that she might have allergic bronchopulmonary aspergillosis. Which one of the following would best help you to confirm your suspicion?

☐ **A** Presence of distal bronchiectasis on CT scan

☐ **B** Improvement occurs following treatment with prednisolone and oral itraconazole

☐ **C** Absence of peripheral eosinophilia

☐ **D** Precipitating antibodies to *Aspergillus fumigatus* antigen

☐ **E** Positive radio-allergo-sorbent test (RAST) to *Aspergillus fumigatus*

3.17   A 32-year-old man with cough and breathlessness is found to have an elevated gas transfer factor on pulmonary function testing. There is a family history of cough and breathlessness. What is the most likely diagnosis?

☐ **A** Pulmonary embolus

☐ **B** Chronic stable asthma

☐ **C** Anaemia of chronic disease

☐ **D** Emphysema due to α_1-antitrypsin deficiency

☐ **E** Extrinsic allergic alveolitis

3.18   You are referred a patient with breathlessness who has previously had a laryngeal carcinoma resected. The ENT surgeon can find no sign of recurrence but can hear some mild inspiratory stridor. Which of the following tests will best help you to decide if there is any element of upper airways (extra-thoracic) obstruction?

☐ **A** Peak expiratory flow rate (PEFR)

☐ **B** Ratio of forced expiratory volume in first second (FEV_1) to forced vital capacity (FVC)

☐ **C** Flow/volume loop

☐ **D** Gas transfer factor

☐ **E** Total lung capacity (TLC)

3.19   A 30-year-old African man is admitted to hospital with fever, cough and night sweats. The admitting team seek your specialist opinion because they think he may have miliary tuberculosis. Which one of the following statements regarding miliary tuberculosis is correct?

☐ **A** A normal chest X-ray excludes the diagnosis

☐ **B** A negative tuberculin test excludes the diagnosis

☐ **C** Anti-TB drugs are not indicated unless sputum is positive for acid-fast bacilli

☐ **D** Nodules are characteristically 3–5 mm in diameter

☐ **E** Tuberculous meningitis co-exists in 15–20% of patients

.20 **A 49-year-old man with a body mass index of 38 kg/m^2 is referred because of snoring. He comes to the clinic with his wife, a GP practice nurse, who tells you that his snoring wakes up the neighbours and that he seems to stop breathing several times per night. She is concerned that he may have obstructive sleep apnoea. Which one of the following features is he least likely to have if his wife has the correct diagnosis?**

☐ **A** Systemic hypertension

☐ **B** Pulmonary hypertension

☐ **C** Difficulty in getting to sleep at night

☐ **D** Polycythaemia

☐ **E** Depression

.21 **A 74-year-old man who has smoked all his life presents with haemoptysis and weight loss. Bronchoscopy reveals the presence of a malignant neoplasm of the lung. Which one of the following is true concerning his possible treatment for his lung cancer?**

☐ **A** Limited-disease small-cell carcinoma should be treated with eight cycles of combination chemotherapy

☐ **B** Adriamycin commonly cause a peripheral neuropathy

☐ **C** In small-cell lung carcinoma mediastinal irradiation should be given before chemotherapy

☐ **D** Hypertrophic pulmonary osteoarthropathy (HPOA) can resolve if the primary tumour is treated

☐ **E** Elderly patients are unable to tolerate chemotherapy or surgery and should receive palliative care only

3.22   A 61-year-old man with an 80 pack/year smoking history is flagged up by
        your radiologist with an abnormal chest X-ray. The patient's GP had sent
        him for this investigation because of chronic cough. The chest X-ray
        shows a mass in the right lower zone and bronchoscopic washings from
        the right lower lobe yields malignant cells. Blood tests are abnormal and
        you consider the possibility of a paraneoplastic phenomenon. Which one
        of the following is true concerning paraneoplastic phenomena?

□   **A**   Paraneoplastic syndromes are caused by metastatic spread of tumour
            to endocrine organs

□   **B**   Eaton–Lambert syndrome occurs most commonly with small-cell
            carcinoma

□   **C**   Desmopressin is used to correct hyponatraemia in the syndrome of
            inappropriate antidiuretic hormone secretion (SIADH)

□   **D**   Hypercalcaemia in lung cancer is most commonly due to ectopic
            parathyroid hormone (PTH) secretion

□   **E**   The presence of a paraneoplastic syndrome is a contraindication to
            surgery

3.23   A 45-year-old woman with breast carcinoma attends the Emergency
        Department with a history of rapid onset of chest pain and breathlessness
        since arriving at Heathrow Airport earlier in the day after a long-haul
        flight back from seeing family in Australia. She is tachypnoeic,
        tachycardic, mildly hypotensive and stable. Which one of the following
        investigations would you perform first to make the diagnosis of
        pulmonary embolism (PE)?

□   **A**   Echocardiography

□   **B**   Leg Doppler ultrasound

□   **C**   Serum D-dimer

□   **D**   CT pulmonary angiogram (spiral CT) scanning

□   **E**   V/Q scanning

.24   **A 60-year-old man with a smoking history of 40/day over many years has a chest X-ray because of breathlessness. This shows a solitary ill-defined mass in the left lower lobe, which on bronchoscopic biopsy turns out to be a squamous cell carcinoma. Which of the following features would render this patient's tumour inoperable?**

☐   **A**   FEV$_1$ of 1.6 litres

☐   **B**   Hypercalcaemia

☐   **C**   Ipsilateral hilar lymph node metastasis

☐   **D**   Ipsilateral supraclavicular lymph node metastasis

☐   **E**   Pleural effusion

Rheumatology and

Immunology

Best of Five

Questions

RHEUMATOLOGY AND IMMUNOLOGY
'BEST OF FIVE' QUESTIONS

For each of the questions select the ONE most appropriate answer from the options provided.

1.1 **An 82-year-old woman presents with non-specific joint pain. She is found to have raised levels of IgM rheumatoid factor (RF) at a titre of 1/64. What is the most appropriate interpretation?**

☐ **A** The presence of rheumatoid factor confirms a diagnosis of rheumatoid arthritis

☐ **B** Carriage of DR4 rheumatoid arthritis-associated alleles is the best predictor of erosive outcome

☐ **C** The prevalence of rheumatoid factor in the elderly is approximately 7%

☐ **D** Raised level of IgM rheumatoid factor suggests that the patient has had a recent infection

☐ **E** Persistence of rheumatoid factor at high titre is a risk factor for the development of rheumatoid arthritis

1.2 **Premature mortality in diffuse systemic sclerosis is most commonly due to:**

☐ **A** Interstital lung disease

☐ **B** Scleroderma renal crisis

☐ **C** Pulmonary hypertension

☐ **D** Cardiovascular disease

☐ **E** Cerebrovascular accidents

Questions: Rheumatology and Immunology

4.3 **A 32-year-old man presents with a history of left-sided knee swelling following an episode of gastroenteritis. In the past he has had episodic low back pain. Which one of the following is the best response?**

- ☐ **A** If he is found to carry the HLA-B27 antigen the course is more likely to be chronic
- ☐ **B** Knee aspiration may reveal the presence of micro-organisms in the joint
- ☐ **C** Absence of conjunctivitis excludes a diagnosis of reactive arthritis
- ☐ **D** Sacro-iliitis is likely to be present on X-rays
- ☐ **E** Antibiotics, if given at an early stage, can limit the extent of joint involvement

4.4 **A 56-year-old woman presents with joint pain, Raynaud's phenomenon and a photosensitive skin rash affecting her face, upper arms and neck. On examination, she is noted to have some proximal muscle weakness. Antinuclear antibody (ANA) is positive and ribonucleoprotein (RNP) antibodies are negative. Which one of the following is the most likely diagnosis?**

- ☐ **A** Systemic lupus erythematosus (SLE)
- ☐ **B** Limited cutaneous systemic sclerosis
- ☐ **C** Dermatomyositis
- ☐ **D** Polymyositis
- ☐ **E** Mixed connective tissue disease

4.5 **A 30-year-old woman with known systemic lupus erythematosus is admitted with fevers, chill and a high temperature. Her disease has been more active recently and she is already on 25 mg prednisolone daily. Which of the following support a flare of disease activity rather than superimposed infection?**

- ☐ **A** Elevated ESR
- ☐ **B** Lymphopenia
- ☐ **C** Elevated gamma glutaryl transferase (GGT)
- ☐ **D** Elevated complement 4
- ☐ **E** Neutrophilia

4.6 **A 72-year-old man presents with a vasculitic skin rash, a peripheral neuropathy and gastrointestinal blood loss. He is found to have proteinuria on dipstick urinalysis. Which one of the following is the most likely diagnosis?**

- ☐ **A** Microscopic polyangiitis
- ☐ **B** Wegener's granulomatosis
- ☐ **C** Henoch–Schönlein vasculitis
- ☐ **D** Polyarteritis nodosa (PAN)
- ☐ **E** Churg–Strauss syndrome

4.7 **A 63-year-old man presents with a 30-year history of nodular rheumatoid arthritis. He has previously received treatment with chloroquine, sulfasalazine, methotrexate and, for at least the last 15 years, with steroids. He has had evidence of poorly controlled inflammation despite these treatments and this has resulted in widespread joint damage. Now he is found to have elevated serum creatinine and proteinuria on urine dipsticks. What would be the most appropriate investigation?**

- ☐ **A** Ultrasound scan of kidneys
- ☐ **B** Renal angiography
- ☐ **C** 24-hour urine collection
- ☐ **D** Gastroscopy
- ☐ **E** Rectal biopsy

4.8 **A 72-year-old man complains of pain around the first metatarsophalangeal (MTP) joint of the left foot. He is otherwise well and is not on any medication. Which one of the following is the best response?**

- ☐ **A** A raised uric acid level would confirm a diagnosis of gout
- ☐ **B** Allopurinol should be commenced if episodes of joint pain are frequent
- ☐ **C** Osteoarthritis (OA) is the most likely diagnosis
- ☐ **D** A normal uric acid excludes a diagnosis of gout
- ☐ **E** Presence of chondrocalcinosis would confirm a diagnosis of pseudogout

4.9 A 65-year-old woman complains of difficulty lifting her arms above her head. Which one of the following is the most useful initial test to aid in diagnosis?

- ☐ **A** Muscle biopsy
- ☐ **B** Erythrocyte sedimentation rate (ESR)
- ☐ **C** Trial of steroids at 1 mg/kg per day
- ☐ **D** Creatinine kinase
- ☐ **E** Temporal artery biopsy

4.10 An 83-year-old woman with mobility problems is started on maintenance treatment with low-dose (7.5 mg/day) oral prednisolone for her rheumatoid arthritis. Which one of the following responses is the best?

- ☐ **A** Routine bone density scanning is not required as osteoprotection should be routinely prescribed in this situation
- ☐ **B** Etidronate should be added to her treatment
- ☐ **C** Routine calcium supplementation is unnecessary
- ☐ **D** When considering treatment decisions, results of bone density should be compared with an age-matched control
- ☐ **E** Osteoporosis is diagnosed when the T score is $\leqslant -2.5$

4.11 A 53-year-old woman complains of her fingers and toes turning white when she is working in the garden. On examination, she is noted to have sclerodactyly, oedema of her fingers and tight skin up to her upper arms. Which one of the following statements is the best response?

- ☐ **A** The diagnosis is limited cutaneous systemic sclerosis (CREST)
- ☐ **B** Treatment with penicillamine can reverse the skin changes
- ☐ **C** Angiotensin-converting enzyme (ACE) inhibitors should be introduced as soon as any rise in blood pressure is noted
- ☐ **D** The most common cause of death is pulmonary hypertension
- ☐ **E** Antinuclear antibody (ANA) may be positive

Answers on pages 125–13

4.12   **Which is the most common presentation of arthritis associated with sarcoidosis?**

☐   **A**   Self-limiting, benign condition principally affecting the lower limbs

☐   **B**   Polyarthritis associated with bilateral hilar lymphadenopathy and erythema marginatum

☐   **C**   Oligoarthritis affecting the lower limbs, associated with bilateral hilar lymphadenopathy and erythema nodosum

☐   **D**   Polyarthritis associated with bilateral hilar lymphadenopathy and erythema nodosum

☐   **E**   Asymmetrical arthritis affecting the large joints of the upper limb and erythema chronicum migrans

4.13   **A young man develops swelling of the distal interphalangeal (DIP) joints of the right middle and little and the left ring fingers. He has had plaque psoriasis since the age of 28 and presents with nail pitting and onycholysis on examination. His IgM rheumatoid factor (RF) titre is positive at 1/32. Select the best response from the following statements:**

☐   **A**   The presence of rheumatoid factor (RF) excludes a diagnosis of psoriatic arthritis

☐   **B**   Arthritis of the distal interphalangeal (DIP) joints is usually associated with nail involvement

☐   **C**   Presence of HLA-B27 would confirm a diagnosis of psoriatic arthritis

☐   **D**   Chronic anterior uveitis is the characteristic ocular manifestation

☐   **E**   Antimalarials are contraindicated as they may exacerbate his skin psoriasis

4.14   **In septic arthritis, the commonest causative micro-organism is which one of the following?**

☐   **A**   *Streptococcus pyogenes*

☐   **B**   *Staphylococcus aureus*

☐   **C**   *Haemophilus influenzae*

☐   **D**   *Borrelia burgdorferi*

☐   **E**   *Neisseria gonorrhoeae*

4.15 **Which one of the following is the characteristic type of eye involvement in juvenile idiopathic arthritis?**

- ☐ **A** Asymptomatic posterior uveitis
- ☐ **B** Bilateral acute anterior uveitis
- ☐ **C** Chronic anterior iridocyclitis
- ☐ **D** Unilateral scleritis
- ☐ **E** Bilateral conjunctivitis

4.16 **A 50-year-old woman presents with knee pain. She is on medication for non-insulin-dependent diabetes mellitus, hypertension and moderate congestive cardiac failure. She has rheumatoid arthritis and is treated with methotrexate and low-dose prednisolone. She is commenced on a nonsteroidal anti-inflammatory drug (NSAID). Which one of the following drugs can interact with the NSAID?**

- ☐ **A** Angiotensin-converting enzyme (ACE) inhibitors
- ☐ **B** Methotrexate
- ☐ **C** Oral hypoglycaemics
- ☐ **D** Thiazide diuretics
- ☐ **E** Any of these items

4.17 **A 72-year-old man presents to the Emergency Department with a low trauma fracture to the wrist following a seizure. He has taken phenytoin for seizures, a β-blocker for hypertension, and prednisolone for polymyalgia rheumatica for many years. He complains of impotence and lethargy. In his history, which one of the following is not suggestive of a risk factor for osteoporosis?**

- ☐ **A** Being male and 72 years of age
- ☐ **B** Impotence
- ☐ **C** Use of a β-blocker
- ☐ **D** Use of corticosteroids
- ☐ **E** Use of phenytoin

Answers on pages 125–13▪

4.18 **Which one of the following statements regarding drug-induced lupus (DIL) is not true?**

- ☐ **A** Central nervous system and renal involvement is uncommon in DIL
- ☐ **B** Classical lupus skin findings (malar rash, oral ulcers, alopecia) are uncommon in DIL
- ☐ **C** Drugs implicated in the aetiology of DIL should not be used in idiopathic systemic lupus erythematosus
- ☐ **D** Methyldopa is implicated in causing DIL
- ☐ **E** More than 50% of patients taking procainamide for more than 12 months develop positive antinuclear antibody titres

4.19 **Antineutrophil cytoplasmic antibodies (ANCA) are associated with which one of the following?**

- ☐ **A** Felty's syndrome
- ☐ **B** Human immunodeficiency virus
- ☐ **C** Inflammatory bowel disease
- ☐ **D** Wegener's granulomatosis
- ☐ **E** All of the options

4.20 **Which one of the following is characteristic of polymyalgia rheumatica?**

- ☐ **A** Inflammatory infiltrates on muscle biopsy
- ☐ **B** An abnormal electromyogram (EMG)
- ☐ **C** High signal seen on T2-weighted MRI scan of the thighs
- ☐ **D** Elevated C-reactive protein (CRP) and a normochromic normocytic anaemia
- ☐ **E** Skip lesions on a biopsy of the temporal artery

4.21 **A recognised complication of long-standing ankylosing spondylitis is:**

- ☐ **A** Aortic stenosis
- ☐ **B** Chronic anterior uveitis
- ☐ **C** Basal lung fibrosis
- ☐ **D** Atlanto-axial subluxation
- ☐ **E** Membranous glomerulonephritis

4.22 A 54-year-old woman presents with joint pain, fatigue and swelling involving the proximal interphalangeal joints of the hands. An X-ray is reported to show ulnar deviation at the metacarpophalangeal joints but no erosions were noted. Which is the most likely diagnosis?

- ☐ **A** Systemic lupus erythematosus
- ☐ **B** Rheumatoid arthritis
- ☐ **C** Osteoarthritis
- ☐ **D** Psoriasis
- ☐ **E** Gout

4.23 A 35-year-old woman is referred from her general practice following a presentation with shortness of breath, myalgia and arthralgia. Laboratory tests for extractable nuclear antigens are positive for anti-Sm, RNP and Ro (SS-A). Which one of the following is the most likely diagnosis?

- ☐ **A** Polymyositis
- ☐ **B** Rheumatoid arthritis
- ☐ **C** Sjögren's syndrome
- ☐ **D** Systemic lupus erythematosus
- ☐ **E** Systemic sclerosis

4.24 Which one of the following is a feature of aggressive disease in rheumatoid arthritis?

- ☐ **A** Functional disability
- ☐ **B** High rheumatoid factor titre
- ☐ **C** Raised C-reactive protein
- ☐ **D** Rheumatoid nodules
- ☐ **E** All of the options

Answers on pages 125–134

4.25 A 58-year-old man presents with blurred vision, an occipital headache, fatigue and shoulder girdle pain. On examination he has scalp tenderness, myalgia but no myopathy, and no evidence of fundoscopic or neurological abnormality. Which one of the following would be the correct immediate action?

☐ **A** Commence a non-steroidal anti-inflammatory drug

☐ **B** Commence oral prednisolone at 20 mg/day

☐ **C** Request an erythrocyte sedimentation rate (ESR) and temporal artery biopsy

☐ **D** Request a computed tomography (CT) scan of the head

☐ **E** Start the patient on 60 mg/day oral prednisolone

4.26 A 34-year-old hiker returned from a 2-week vacation in the American Great Lakes 4 weeks ago. He complains of a flitting arthralgia, myalgia, bone pain and a swollen knee. He recalls an episode lasting several days on vacation where he had a headache, irritated eyes, a sore throat and swollen glands, and he has a persistent rash. He denies sexual contact. Which one of the following would be the most useful diagnostic test?

☐ **A** Aspirate and culture the knee effusion for gonococcal infection

☐ **B** Biopsy the rash or a palpable lymph node

☐ **C** Measure serum antinuclear antibodies

☐ **D** Measure spirochaete antibodies

☐ **E** Measure the serum antistreptolysin-O antibody titre (ASOT)

4.27 A 30-year-old woman collapses at her GP surgery. On arrival in the Emergency Department she is short of breath and hypoxic, with pleuritic sounding chest pain. The patient is able to confirm that she is already on warfarin following a similar episode a year ago and that she lost a pregnancy in the first 3 months just 2 years ago. There is a family history of arthritis and her sister takes medication for a kidney disease. Which one of the following statements is the least correct in this scenario?

☐ **A** A dsDNA antibody titre could be useful

☐ **B** Sudden widespread organ failure may occur

☐ **C** There is a risk of arterial as well as venous thrombosis

☐ **D** Thrombocytopenia may be present

☐ **E** Warfarin should be dosed to maintain the INR at 2.0

4.28 **Which one of the following is a recognised cause of ectopic calcification?**

☐ **A** Dermatomyositis

☐ **B** Hypoparathyroidism

☐ **C** Chondrocalcinosis

☐ **D** Systemic lupus erythematosus

☐ **E** Hypothyroidism

4.29 **HLA-B27**

☐ **A** Is found in up to 30% of the normal population

☐ **B** Is found in over 90% patients with ankylosing spondylitis world-wide

☐ **C** Is associated with osteitis condensans ilii in which the sacro-iliac joints are affected

☐ **D** Is associated with chronic anterior uveitis

☐ **E** Is associated with acute anterior uveitis independently of systemic joint disease

4.30 **A young man is diagnosed as having pseudohypoparathyroidism. Which one of the following laboratory tests is consistent with this diagnosis?**

☐ **A** Low parathyroid levels

☐ **B** Hypercalcaemia

☐ **C** Hypophosphataemia

☐ **D** None of these items

☐ **E** Raised parathyroid hormone

Answers on pages 125–134

ANSWERS

Cardiology

CARDIOLOGY: 'BEST OF FIVE' ANSWERS

1.1   E: VVI pacing

In the jugular venous pressure waveform the *a*-wave corresponds to atrial contraction; the *v*-wave is caused by the final phase of atrial filling; and the descending limb of the *v*-wave (the *y*-descent) is caused by ventricular filling as the tricuspid valve opens. In contrast to the physiological state, in tricuspid regurgitation the *v*-wave corresponds to ventricular contraction and therefore occurs simultaneously with the carotid pulse. As such, it truly represents a *cv*-wave. Cannon waves are due to simultaneous ventricular and atrial contraction and may occur with VVI pacing (if independent atrial activity is present), complete heart block and ventricular tachycardia. The associated rise in left atrial pressure and reduction in ventricular filling is the cause of the pacemaker syndrome. Constrictive and restrictive cardiac disease, along with tamponade, cause paradoxical increase in jugular venous pressure on inspiration. In atrial fibrillation the *a*-wave is lost and in flutter *f*-waves are seen. As the patient is well, VT and pacemaker failure are extremely unlikely as before pacing the patient felt symptomatic.

1.2   B: Angiotensin-converting enzyme (ACE) inhibitor

While all of these agents are effective antihypertensives, an ACE inhibitor would be the optimal initial option in a patient with prior coronary artery bypass grafting (CABG). In addition to their beneficial effects on blood pressure reduction, ACE inhibitors appear to have additional benefits in patients with evidence of significant vascular disease, irrespective of left ventricular function. The HOPE study demonstrated that treatment with ramipril reduced the rates of death, myocardial infarction and stroke to an extent that could not be accounted for by blood pressure reduction alone. This study included patients with known angina, previous unstable angina, percutaneous coronary inter-vention and CABG. The 2006 *NICE Hypertension Guidelines* state that White patients under the age of 55 should initially be treated with an ACE inhibitor. Afro-Caribbean patients (who have lower levels of renin) and those aged over 55 should initially be treated with a calcium-channel blocker or a diuretic. Many patients require at least dual therapy to obtain adequate control.

1.3   A: Intravenous β-blocker

Aortic dissection can be subdivided depending upon the site of origin of the dissection flap. Type A involves the ascending aorta (approximately 65%) and type B begins distal to the ascending aorta, usually just after the origin of the left subclavian artery. Management of these two presentations is very different.

Type B dissections are generally treated medically, with aggressive control of blood pressure in an attempt to reduce complications. Surgical intervention is extremely difficult and carries a significant risk of paraplegia. This is therefore usually reserved for patients with complications such as aortic rupture, vital organ or limb ischaemia or unremitting pain. However, endovascular repair is currently being tried in several specialised centres and this may provide a future alternative therapy. Early surgical intervention is indicated in the case of type A dissection and involves replacement of the diseased part of the aortic root and then re-establishing aortic continuity using a prosthetic graft. Precise blood pressure control is also mandatory in this setting. To optimise blood pressure control an intravenous agent with a short half-life is preferred. Ideally if not contraindicated, this would be in the form of a β-blocker such as propranolol or labetalol (α- and β-receptor blocker), which have beneficial effects on arterial wall stress by reducing arterial dP/dt (rate of change of arterial wall pressure). If β-blockers were contraindicated then appropriate intravenous alternatives would include nitroprusside or GTN. Oral agents can also be added and calcium-channel blockers reduce both arterial pressure and arterial dP/dt.

1.4   A: Call for help

The 2005 *Guidelines* state that the first step is to call for help. CPR should then begin at a rate of 30 compressions to two breaths until a defibrillator with monitor arrives to determine whether he has a shockable rhythm (pulseless ventricular tachycardia or ventricular fibrillation). Note the previous recommendation of two rescue breaths has been removed. See Resuscitation Guidelines 2005 http://www.resus.org.uk

1.5   E: 150 J biphasic shock

On identifying a shockable rhythm the next step is to deliver an appropriate shock. The first shock should be at least 150 J with a biphasic machine or 360 with a monophasic machine. Intubation may subsequently be carried out during CPR. CPR should be continued for a further 2 minutes even if the patient has been defibrillated back to sinus rhythm. In ongoing arrest scenario adrenaline should be given every 2 to 3 minutes.

1.6   B: Candesartan

Spironolactone was found to reduce mortality in hospitalized patients with class III or IV heart failure. Spironolactone should not be prescribed without specialist advice in patients with a serum creatinine over 220 mmol/l due to the risk of hyperkalaemia. Eplerenone currently has a license for early post-MI heart failure, following the EPHESUS trial, a randomized placebo controlled trial of eplerenone in patients with left ventricular failure post-MI with an ejection fraction of 40% or less. All patients on aldosterone antagonists require monitoring of potassium level. As this patient is not in pulmonary oedema, but in NYHA class II, then an aldosterone antagonist is not indicated by current clinical trial evidence. Digoxin may reduce hospitalisations for heart failure, but has no effect on mortality, although withdrawal of digoxin in patients already established on this therapy has been associated with an increase in mortality. Currently, it is uncommon to add digoxin to patients unless in atrial fibrillation with heart failure or severe resistant symptoms. Angiotensin II antagonists (AIIA) may be used in addition to an ACE inhibitor (ACEI). Candesartan is licensed for this purpose in the UK following the CHARM study. Adding an AIIA to β-blockers and ACEI resulted in a significant 15% relative risk reduction of cardiovascular death or admission to hospital for worsening chronic heart failure and so this combination may be considered, again with appropriate biochemistry monitoring.

.7   C: Clopidogrel 600 mg and transfer for primary percutaneous coronary intervention (travelling time to centre 1 hour)

Comparison studies suggest similar mortality outcomes for thrombolysis and primary percutaneous coronary intervention (PPCI – acute infarct angioplasty) within the first 2 hours of the onset of symptoms of acute myocardial infarction. After 2 hours, despite the additional transfer time, morbidity and mortality are reduced by PPCI. Currently, clopidogrel 600 mg is given before any PCI, unless the patients have been established on clopidogrel for over 1 week. Streptokinase is less effective than other thrombolytics in terms of vessel patency and anterior myocardial infarcts do better with fibrin specific thrombolytics (eg tenecteplase) if given within 6 hours of onset. As such, tenecteplase would be a viable option if PPCI was unavailable. Clopidogrel was given as 75 mg within 24 hours of ST elevation myocardial infarction in the Commit – CCS2 trial. The addition of clopidogrel to thrombolysis and aspirin showed a 7% relative risk reduction of in-hospital mortality. Clopidogrel was given as 300 mg within 12 hours of MI in the CLARITY trial that looked at artery patency at angiography after thrombolysis in patients under 75 years. The addition of clopidogrel to aspirin and thrombolysis resulted in an absolute risk reduction of 2.5% of the composite of death, MI and recurrent ischaemia requiring revascularisation at 30 days.

1.8   A: Cardiac amyloidosis

Cardiac amyloidosis results in a typical echocardiographic appearance of LVH, thickened intra-atrial septum and valvular leaflets. Left ventricular function is often impaired despite normal left ventricular cavity size due to failure of systolic thickening. The electrocardiogram (ECG) shows small complexes and this provides a clue to the diagnosis in the face of LVH. Diagnostic tests include serum amyloid protein scans, cardiac magnetic resonance imaging, serum light chain assessment and biopsy of rectum/intra-abdominal fat to confirm the presence of amyloid. Amyloidosis may be treated if diagnosed early. Severe amyloidosis causes severe heart failure and the terminal stage is often marked by syncope. Hypertension, aortic stenosis and hypertrophic cardiomyopathy may result in LVH on both ECG and ECHO. Haemochromatosis results in impairment of left ventricular function and should be suspected in patients with impaired LV function, hyperpigmentation and diabetes ('bronze' diabetes). Haemochromatosis does not usually result in voltage criteria for LVH on the ECG.

1.9   A: Cardiac resynchronisation pacemaker

This patient has left bundle branch block, which will cause intra-ventricular and inter-ventricular desynchrony. Left bundle branch block is associated with cardiac failure. This patient meets the electrocardiogram (ECG) and clinical criteria for response to cardiac resynchronisation pacing (CRT-P). CRT-P involves pacing both ventricles together, with the left ventricular lead passed into the coronary sinus into a distant vein. CRT-P has been shown to reduce symptoms of heart failure and pooled results from CARE-HF and COMPANION involving 2333 patients found a reduction in mortality from heart failure (HR 0.61, 95% CI 0.44 to 0.83). The ECG criteria are first-degree arteriovenous (AV) block and left bundle branch block and the clinical criteria are New York Hospital Association class III (symptoms on minimal exertion) or IV (symptoms at rest) heart failure. CRT-P should be considered once patients are taking optimum medical heart failure therapy. Cardiac resynchronisation pacing (without implantable cardioverter defibrillator (ICD)) reduced the absolute risk of sudden cardiac death by 10% in the CARE-HF trial. Patients with class III and IV heart failure should be assessed for CRT once on maximal medical therapy. Patients with severe end stage heart failure (class IV) should not receive an implantable cardioverter defibrillator unless the heart failure improves or they are awaiting transplantation. Although cardiac transplantation is one of the great successes of 21st century medicine, only a limited number are performed due to organ shortage. The use of CRT may avoid the need for transplantation. Left ventricular assist devices (LVAD) are currently implanted

Answers: Cardiology

as a bridge to transplantation or to allow a heart to recover from a reversible insult (eg fulminant myocarditis) in a critically unwell patient. The use of LVADs without a further treatment available is currently not widespread practice, although is an area of active interest for transplant centres.

.10   E: Ramipril 1.25 mg bd + eplerenone 25 mg od

Eplerenone has been shown to reduce the relative risk of cardiac mortality and hospitalisation for cardiovascular events of patients with heart failure after MI by 13% in the EPHESUS study. Multiple randomized placebo-controlled trials have shown that ACEI reduce mortality after MI, particularly in patients with left ventricular impairment. β-Blockers reduce mortality after MI particularly in patients with heart failure, but are contraindicated in acute pulmonary oedema. Once the pulmonary oedema has cleared these patients should receive β-blocker therapy, as patients who have impaired left ventricular function receive the highest absolute benefit. Intravenous GTN is a very effective initial treatment of acute pulmonary oedema.

.11   E: Intra-aortic balloon pump (IABP) insertion and trial of sodium nitroprusside

This patient is at extremely high risk of death and aortic valve replacement is extremely high risk in the presence of pulmonary oedema. Early liaison with cardiothoracic surgeons is vital to decide timing of AVR. Urgent IABP insertion may be life saving in this situation and providing there are no contraindications should proceed immediately. IABP insertion is via the femoral artery with the balloon placed in the descending aorta; inflation during diastole augments coronary, cerebral and renal perfusion as well as decreasing after load by deflating during systole. Sodium nitroprusside is a powerful arterial and venous dilator and is indicated for treatment of patients with decompensated heart failure, impaired left ventricular function and aortic stenosis.

.12   A: Clopidogrel 600 mg + primary PCI + IABP insertion

This patient is in cardiogenic shock due to an acute myocardial infarction. The best treatment is primary percutaneous coronary intervention (PPCI) with intra-aortic balloon pump (IABP) support. Thrombolysis is likely to be ineffective due to the hypotension. Clopidogrel is given as 600 mg before PCI.

1.13   A: Cardiac magnetic resonance imaging

The underlying diagnosis is likely to be arrhythmogenic right ventricular cardiomyopathy. This is an autosomal dominant disorder, with a penetrance of 20–30%. The age at presentation is usually 20–30 years. There may be a family history of sudden cardiac death (SCD); it is the second commonest diagnosed cause of SCD in young people after hypertrophic cardiomyopathy. Palpitations, syncope, aborted sudden cardiac death and fatigue are the most common presenting features. Young patients may have reduced exercise tolerance or dizzy spells during exertion as VT is often precipitated by catecholaminergic drive. There is no genetic test for this condition. Diagnosis is made based on family history, examination, electrocardiogram (ECG) abnormalities, echocardiogram findings of an abnormal and often dilated right heart. Fibro-fatty replacement of the myocardium may be detected at cardiac magnetic resonance imaging. This investigation is routine in the assessment of such a patient. Other tests include a right ventricular angiogram and right ventricular myocardial biopsy.

1.14   E: Trans-oesophageal echocardiography and, if satisfactory, proceed to DC cardioversion

The ventricular response in atrial flutter is often difficult to control with arteriovenous (AV) node blocking medications and chemical cardioversion is usually unsuccessful. A trans-oesophageal echocardiogram (TOE) will show whether there is a clot in the left atrial appendage – if not then immediate cardioversion followed by warfarinisation for a minimum of 6 weeks is appropriate. Recurrent atrial flutter may be treated by atrial flutter ablation (an electrophysiology technique). It is not safe to cardiovert patients who have not been treated with anticoagulants and whose onset of the flutter is greater than 48 hours due to the risk of embolic stroke unless a TOE has shown a clean left atrial appendage.

1.15   A: Anderson–Fabry disease

This is a rare disease (1/40,000) caused by lack of the α-galactosidase A enzyme (α-Gal A) due to mutations in the *Gal* gene at Xq22. As a result there is intra-lysosomal accumulation of glycosphingolipids. The clinical features include pain, a characteristic rash called angiokeratoma corporis diffusum, left ventricular hypertrophy, stroke at a young age and renal failure. Recently, a recombinant replacement therapy became available. Burgada syndrome consists of characteristic electrocardiogram (ECG) abnormalities (cove ST elevation in the anterior leads) with a high risk of sudden cardiac death. Burgada is usually due to a mutation of the sodium channel (SNC5A) and may be

Answers: Cardiology

1.16   E: Temporary pacing

Torsades de pointes is a polymorphic ventricular tachycardia, which is often related to significant QT interval prolongation. Prevention of Torsades de pointes requires removal of precipitants, which includes amiodarone and correcting hypokalaemia and hypomagnesiumaemia. Intravenous magnesium should be administered, even if plasma levels are within the normal range, as plasma levels correlate poorly with intracellular levels. Temporary pacing at a relatively fast rate such as 80 to 90 shortens the QT interval and is often very successful, particularly with concomitant β-blockade.

1.17   B: Fractured pacing lead

Pacing at the right ventricular apex results in a left bundle branch block pattern. Pacing of the left ventricle results in a RBBB pattern. The coronary sinus is used to access lateral cardiac veins to pace the left ventricle in patients who have biventricular pacemakers. Coronary sinus pacing was used in the past to pace the left atrium. It is important to examine the electrocardiogram (ECG) of the patient while pacing to ensure the lead is in the correct position. It is unusual nowadays to see perforation of the right ventricle with permanent leads. The fact that there was RBBB during pacing is indicative of the lead pacing the left ventricle. A patent foramen ovale (PFO) is seen in up to 20% of the population and cases of stroke due to thrombus on the pacing lead sited in the left ventricle having passed through a PFO are well reported. Subclavian vein thrombosis is unlikely to cause a stroke, although passage of a thrombus via a PFO is possible. Tricuspid valve endocarditis will cause septic embolisation to the lungs, but unless there is a co-existent arteriovenous (AV) malformation within the lungs a stroke is impossible.

1.18   D: Trans-oesophageal echocardiogram

A lengthening PR interval is of concern as the arteriovenous (AV) node lies close to the aortic valve suggesting an aortic valve abscess, which can only be treated with urgent valve replacement surgery. In this case, the C-reactive protein (CRP) was misleading and so must always be interpreted in the clinical context. A radiolabelled white cell scan is less straightforward to arrange and is likely to take longer than a TOE and will not directly visualise the area of concern. Inserting any form of permanent pacemaker should be avoided if there is concern of ongoing infection.

1.19   C: Digoxin

In this case an echocardiogram is not available, so the safest option is to avoid negatively inotropic medications and treat with digoxin. β-Blockers are contra-indicated in patients with decompensated heart failure due to impaired left ventricular (LV) function, but once out of pulmonary oedema β-blockers would be an attractive option. Verapamil is contraindicated in patients with LV impairment. Flecainide is negatively inotropic and is contraindicated in struc-tural heart disease. Oral amiodarone will take too long to accumulate to have effect.

1.20   E: Radiofrequency atrial fibrillation (AF) ablation

Implantable atrial defibrillators have largely been unpopular with patients. Atrial fibrillation suppression algorithms on pacemakers are generally unsuc-cessful at preventing AF, apart from patients with sinus node disease where there is evidence of benefit. However, once the arteriovenous (AV) node is ablated the pacemaker can be programmed to 'mode switch', ie to pace the ventricle after the atrial depolarisation when in sinus rhythm, but once in AF to provide back up ventricular pacing independent of atrial activity. Amiodarone has multiple side-effects, including epidimo-orchitis which risks infertility, so would best be avoided, especially in a 35-year-old man. AF surgery would usually be reserved for patients with intractable symptoms where AF ablation has failed. AV node ablation and PPM insertion results in pacemaker depen-dency so again is best avoided in a patient aged 35. AF ablation is a relatively new procedure and is indicated in patients with intractable PAF symptoms who have found drug therapy ineffective. AF ablation is a percutaneous technique with access from the femoral veins. Currently, the risk of serious complication is quoted at 1% (pulmonary vein stenosis, tamponade, oesophageal fistula) and around 20% of patients need more than one procedure. To access the left atrium a trans-septal puncture is made and then parts of the left atrium and the pulmonary veins are ablated.

1.21   C: Pericardial tamponade

The signs are consistent with tamponade, which will be released by opening the chest and will allow the source of bleeding to be determined. Pericardial tamponade is not uncommon in the immediate postoperative period. Pulmon-ary embolism is unlikely as patients are fully heparinised while on bypass and the time period is too early. Constrictive pericarditis would not occur this early. A gastrointestinal (GI) bleed would result in a lower CVP rather than a high one. Right ventricular infarction is possible (due to air embolism or thrombus embolism) but is much less likely than pericardial tamponade.

.22   A: Bisoprolol

Pregnancy is a risk factor for aortic rupture in patients with Marfan's syndrome, so ideally patients should be able to go through the implications of pregnancy preconception to decide how to proceed. Patients with enlarged aortic roots or whose aortic root is enlarging on serial measurements may require elective aortic arch replacement before pregnancy. β-Blockers have been shown to reduce the risk of aortic rupture by reducing shear stress. However, careful counselling is required before prescribing any medication in women of child-bearing age. β-Blockers are associated with intra-uterine growth retardation so must be used with caution in pregnancy. There is no evidence that methyl-dopa or sotalol are helpful and ramipril should be avoided as it is not known to be helpful and is also harmful to a fetus.

.23   A: Acute stent thrombosis

Stent thrombosis is the most likely cause of the sudden deterioration. Left ventricular scarring tends to occur later, once fibrosis has occurred. Peri-infarct arrhythmias occur in the context of vessel occlusion and reperfusion within the first 48 hours. Idiopathic VF is defined as occurring when other causes have been excluded.

.24   D: Implantable loop recorder insertion

The *European Syncope Guidelines* currently recommend this approach in patients who have electrocardiogram (ECG) abnormalities suggestive of an arrhythmia, but no positive evidence. Electrophysiological studies have not been shown to be cost-effective for this indication. Carotid sinus syndrome is unlikely to have been the cause of this patient's syncope. Tilt testing is unlikely to be rewarding as the episodes occurred at rest.

.25   B: MR renal angiogram

The history of flash pulmonary oedema is without obvious cardiac cause. Renal artery stenosis is a well recognised cause. Renal artery stenosis should be considered as the most likely diagnosis since the history is of hypertension, chronic renal impairment with asymmetrical kidney sizes on ultrasound and evidence of vascular disease (femoral bruit). MRA is the first line investigation and if renal artery stenosis is confirmed angioplasty should be considered. An implantable loop recorder is a very useful way of obtaining a diagnosis for patients with intermittent arrhythmias or unexplained syncope.

1.26   D: Flecainide challenge

The suspicion from the history is of an inherited channelopathy, such as long QT or Burgada syndrome. Burgada syndrome is a sodium channelopathy and is common is patients from Thailand. In patients with non-diagnostic ECGs it may be unmasked by an infusion of flecainide, which may reveal the characteristic cove ST elevation in the precordial leads. Examination of a heart at post mortem is usually normal and hence a CMR is likely to be normal. Carotid sinus massage and tilt tests are unhelpful.

1.27   E: Rescue angioplasty

This patient is in cardiogenic shock and the evidence from the SHOCK trial shows that revascularisation within the first 24 hours, with intra-aortic balloon pump support reduces mortality in patients aged less than 75 years. Evidence from the REACT trial found that re-thrombolysis increases bleeding complications with no mortality benefit. This patient is already well filled, as evidenced by the pulmonary capillary wedge pressure (PCWP), which in a patient like this should be maintained at 15 to 20 mmHg. PCWP is helpful in patients with inferior myocardial infarction and shock as residual volume (RV) infarction may occur and therefore right atrial pressure may not accurately reflect left atrial filling. In this setting intravenous fluids may be administered, but where there is doubt about the fluid status the PCWP is helpful. Furosemide will not be helpful in this situation.

1.28   C: Development of atrial fibrillation

Mitral stenosis is unlikely to rapidly progress and cause acute deterioration. The most likely cause of deterioration is development of atrial fibrillation. This results in reduced left ventricular filling due to loss of atrial systole. When the heart rate increases cardiac output decreases, with back pressure into the left atrium (reduced diastolic filling time) resulting in pulmonary oedema and pulmonary hypertension. The priority in this patient is to control the heart rate and anticoagulate (high stroke risk), and consideration will need to be given to mitral valve intervention.

Answers: Cardiology

.29   B: Bisoprolol and warfarin

With intermittent atrial fibrillation, ischaemic heart disease and impaired ventricular function, this man will benefit from full anticoagulation to reduce stroke risk. With impaired ventricular function and ischaemic heart disease he will benefit prognostically from β-blockade. Although amiodarone is an acceptable answer from the anti-arrhythmic perspective it ignores the prognostic benefit this man will derive from β-blockade and is not offered as an answer in conjunction with anticoagulation. Flecainide and sotalol are associated with excess mortality in patients with ischaemia or heart failure. Digoxin limits ventricular rate in sustained AF but has previously been shown to increase paroxysmal AF.

.30   D: Troponin I level

A plasma troponin I measured 12 hours after symptoms would be extremely helpful in determining this patient's initial management. If this is negative and the electrocardiogram (ECG) normal, then it is safe to send the patient home and arrange further investigations as an out-patient, if required. Plasma levels of troponin I are highly specific for myocardial damage and, in particular, a normal level measured at 12 hours has a very high negative predictive value for adverse cardiac events in the context of a normal ECG. Plasma levels can, however, be elevated in other conditions such as renal failure; in this group of patients paired measurements are helpful (there should be a rise and fall if there is myocardial damage). Although an exercise test would also help clarify diagnosis and subsequent risk, this should not be performed until cardiac biomarkers have excluded an acute cardiac event in patients presenting with significant chest pain. Clearly, if diagnostic doubt still exists, an exercise test is positive or the troponin is elevated angiography would be warranted.

.31   C: Primary percutaneous coronary intervention with temporary wire cover

Although this woman has developed CHB she is haemodynamically stable, without clinical evidence of pulmonary oedema. This has occurred in the context of an acute inferior infarction, primarily because the right coronary artery contributes to the blood supply of the atrioventricular (AV) node (via the AV nodal branch). In acute myocardial infarction early restoration of coronary artery blood flow has a major influence on prognosis. In a 70-year-old woman with an inferior infarct this would ideally be attempted with primary percutaneous coronary intervention (PCI). Primary PCI has a mortality benefit over thrombolysis if it can be delivered within 90 minutes of diagnosis of acute MI. Although temporary pacing has not been shown to improve prognosis in acute

MI, it should be used in patients with inferior infarction and CHB with evidence of haemodynamic compromise. Patients presenting with CHB in the context of an anterior infarct have a particularly poor prognosis, primarily due to the extensive amount of damaged myocardium. In this situation temporary pacing should be routinely used to try to prevent bradycardia-associated hypotension and the increased risk of ventricular asystole associated with this presentation. Thrombolysis should not be delayed if this is the strategy that has been chosen to reperfuse the myocardium. Then pacing can be performed via the femoral veins or where available a pacing wire is placed at the same time as gaining arterial access for primary PCI.

1.32   C: Presence of co-existing coronary artery disease

Symptomatic aortic stenosis is an indication for surgery (unless determined inappropriate for other medical reasons). Trans-thoracic echocardiography can provide accurate details of peak aortic valve gradient together with estimates of left ventricular function. Patients with evidence of left ventricular dysfunction even if severe, should still undergo assessment for valve replacement since function may significantly improve post-operatively and prognosis without surgery is particularly poor. Remember, the peak gradient will be reduced when left ventricular function is impaired. The aortic valve area can be calculated at echocardiography, although it must be interpreted with caution as it relies on precise measurements and, as such, errors may occur. In patients with impaired left ventricular function modest aortic valve gradients may be indicative of severe aortic stenosis. It is, however, important to know the coronary anatomy in the majority of cases: this will determine the requirement for concomitant coronary artery bypass grafting and peri-operative risk. Right heart pressures will not influence the need for surgical intervention and although there may be co-existent aortic incompetence there is no doubt in this case that valve replacement is required.

1.33   A: Addition of β-blocker

There is now considerable evidence to support the use of β-blockers in the treatment of chronic heart failure for patients in either sinus rhythm or AF (COPERNICUS – carvedilol, CBIS-II – bisoprolol, MERIT-HF – metoprolol controlled release). Although digoxin is usually effective in controlling resting heart rates it less effective during exercise. β-Blockers are, however, particularly useful in this setting. AV node ablation and pacemaker insertion is an irreversible intervention and should be reserved for patients intolerant of medication or in whom it is ineffective despite adequate dosing. AF can be paroxysmal, persistent (but possibly amenable to cardioversion) or permanent. By definition, permanent AF cannot be converted to sinus rhythm.

.34   C: Radiofrequency ablation of the accessory pathway

The history is suggestive of paroxysmal tachycardia in the context of WPW. Most supra-ventricular tachycardias presenting to hospital are nodal (ie atrioventricular (AV) nodal tachycardias), but patients with WPW have an extra pathway connecting the atria to the ventricle (an AV re-entrant tachycardia). In WPW, the ventricular response during AF can be extremely rapid as a result of anterograde conduction down the accessory pathway. This can degenerate into ventricular fibrillation. In this young, symptomatic patient radiofrequency ablation of the accessory pathway is a potentially curative procedure that can be carried out with minimal risk. Patients who present with AF and WPW should undergo in-patient ablation because of the risk of death (NICE, 2006). Although treatment with amiodarone, flecainide or sotalol might be effective in reducing or even abolishing symptoms, therapy would need to be maintained long term.

.35   B: Constrictive pericarditis

In constrictive pericarditis the heavily fibrosed or calcified pericardium restricts diastolic filling of all four chambers of the heart. Patients often present with dyspnoea and fatigue together with symptoms and signs of marked fluid retention. In this case pericardial constriction could be a result of previous tuberculous pericarditis or be secondary to radiotherapy. Examination of the JVP can be very helpful in the clinical assessment of pericardial disease. In constrictive pericarditis there is a rapid *y*, since the majority of ventricular filling occurs in early diastole. Kussmaul's sign (an increase in systemic venous pressure during inspiration) is also seen and results from a failure of transmission of the intrathoracic pressure changes to the pericardial space, seen during normal respiration. In cardiac tamponade the *y*-descent is often absent or blunted. Severe tricuspid incompetence is associated with giant *cv*-waves whereas in superior vena cava obstruction the JVP is elevated and fixed. Patients with tamponade typically demonstrate a significant degree of pulsus paradoxus (>10 mmHg), whereas in those with constriction this tends to occur to a lesser degree (<10 mmHg).

.36   B: ASD – ostium secundum

The results show normal aortic and wedge pressures but slightly elevated right heart pressures. A step-up in saturation is seen at the level of the right atrium, thereby demonstrating the presence of a left-to-right shunt at this level and so confirming the diagnosis of an atrial septal defect. Secundum defects are the most common (approximately 70%) and often remain asymptomatic until the fourth and fifth decades when patients may present with atrial arrhythmias (although exact timing and nature of presentation will be dependent upon the size of the shunt). Primum defects are usually detected earlier in life due to associated mitral and tricuspid valve defects. Sinus venosus defects are less common (approximately 10–15%) and occur in the upper septum where they may be associated with anomalous pulmonary drainage into the right atrium.

1.37   E: Trans-oesophageal echo and early referral for mitral valve replacement

A lengthening PR interval is of concern as the AV node lies close to the aortic valve suggesting an aortic valve abscess, which can only be treated with urgent valve replacement surgery. In this case, the C-reactive protein (CRP) was misleading and so must always be interpreted in the clinical context. A radiolabelled white cell scan is less straightforward to arrange and is likely to take longer than a TOE and will not directly visualise the area of concern. Inserting any form of permanent pacemaker should be avoided if there is concern of ongoing infection.

1.38   A: Dobutamine

This patient has an elevated PCWP, an impaired CI (cardiac output corrected for body surface area) and high SVR (evidence of peripheral vasoconstriction in an attempt to maintain blood pressure). Cardiogenic shock has developed as a result of extensive myocardial damage and hence inotropic support is required. Intravenous fluids should be avoided in view of the elevated PCWP (effectively left atrial pressure). Although iv GTN might be helpful in reducing pulmonary oedema (due to its vasodilatory effects), it would also adversely lower the systemic blood pressure in this case. Dobutamine, a β-receptor agonist, would be the optimum initial drug therapy since it is not only able to increase cardiac output (positive inotropic effects) but also results in a reduction in SVR (decrease in afterload). In contrast, noradrenaline, predominantly an α-receptor agonist, will result in further increases in SVR and therefore increases myocardial oxygen demand due to the increase in afterload. It is, however, the inotropic agent of choice for the management of septic shock where patients have marked vasodilatation. Dopamine (α-, β- and dopaminergic receptor agonist) is a relatively weak positive inotrope and at higher doses results in increased SVR. It is often used at low ('renal') dose in conjunction with other inotropes in an attempt to enhance renal perfusion (by renal vasodilatation and subsequent diuresis, although direct evidence supporting a positive effect on survival is lacking. In this case an intra-aortic balloon pump should be inserted, followed by rescue PCI. Dobutamine should be given while this is being organised.

.39   E: Thrombolysis with tissue plasminogen activator

This patient has clinical features consistent with a haemodynamically compromising pulmonary embolus despite the initiation of LMWH therapy. Thrombolysis is indicated for patients with a proven pulmonary embolus who have evidence of haemodynamic compromise. Tissue plasminogen activator works faster than streptokinase and hence achieves re-perfusion more rapidly and is the preferred choice. Streptokinase can cause hypotension. In patients with severe haemodynamic impairment, additional support with inotropes may also be required, together with cautious iv fluids (eg 500 ml). Whether thrombolysis is indicated in all patients with pulmonary emboli and right heart dilatation (usually diagnosed from echo) has yet to be confirmed. Inferior vena cava filters are reserved for short-term use in patients with proved lower limb deep vein thrombosis (DVT) and evidence of pulmonary emboli, in whom anticoagulation is contraindicated.

.40   D: *Staphylococcus epidermidis*

In the UK, *S. viridans* remain the commonest cause of native valve endocarditis. However, in the first year after valvular surgery the spectrum of infecting organisms is somewhat different, with coagulase-negative staphylococci being the most common (approximately 50%). When individual species are considered, the majority of these are *S. epidermidis.* It is presumed that these infections are nosocomial and, despite the delayed presentation, in many cases are derived from events occurring during the surgical admission. *S. aureus* is a virulent organism and systemic infections often run a fulminant course. Patients with SBE secondary to *S. aureus* are often exceedingly unwell with a relatively short history of illness. *Candida* infection is seen most commonly in intravenous drug abusers.

.41   E: Simvastatin

The greatest evidence for the benefits for lipid lowering in primary prevention comes from studies involving statins. While benefit may also occur for other therapies without adverse effects, this is not entirely clear at present. Two major placebo-controlled statin studies have been performed, evaluating their role in primary prevention. WOSCOPS, using pravastatin, demonstrated a reduction in all-cause mortality of 22% and coronary heart disease incidence by 31% in men aged 45–64 years old and an average cholesterol of 7 mmol/l a randomisation. The AFCAPS/TEXCAPS study evaluated the effect of lovastati in healthy men and women with a mean cholesterol of 5.7 mmol/l an demonstrated a reduction in the incidence of major acute coronary hea disease events of 37%. Omega-3 fish oils have been shown to reduce th incidence of ventricular arrhythmias in patients who have had an anteric myocardial infarction.

1.42   B: Intravenous amiodarone

The differential diagnosis of broad-complex tachycardia includes ventricula tachycardia (VT) or supraventricular tachycardia (SVT) with aberrant conduc tion. While there are many electrocardiogram (ECG) features that can help t differentiate between these two arrhythmias, if any doubt exists it should b treated as per VT. The presence of ischaemic heart disease or known impai ment of ventricular function significantly favours VT. Although this patient currently haemodynamically stable it is important to treat the arrhythm aggressively since decompensation can occur rapidly, particularly with a pric history of myocardial infarction. Although oral amiodarone would be a appropriate option oral loading takes a long time to achieve therapeutic level Overdrive pacing is usually reserved for resistant cases of VT. Trans-oesoph. geal echo can be used to exclude left atrial thrombus before elective cardiove sion. If intravenous amiodarone proved ineffective then early DC cardioversic should be performed.

1.43   E: Thrombus in the left atrial appendage

Percutaneous trans-septal mitral valvuloplasty can be extremely effective treating symptomatic mitral stenosis. In addition, it may result in a decrease previously elevated right heart pressures. Best results are seen in patients wi pure mitral stenosis without valvular calcification and in younger subjec where the sub-valvular chordae have not become thickened and fuse Relative contraindications to this approach include significant mitral regurgit. tion (which may be worsened by the procedure), a rigid, calcified valve an the presence of left atrial thrombus (usually visualised on TOE). While atri fibrillation and spontaneous contrast in the left atrium (seen on echo 'swirling smoke' and thought to reflect sluggish blood flow) are associated wi increased risk of left atrial thrombus formation, on their own they would ne preclude intervention. Patients with thrombus in the left atrial appendag should not undergo percutaneous mitral valvuloplasty.

.44   D: Reverse splitting of the second heart sound

Although the presence of LBBB on the resting electrocardiogram (ECG) is commonly associated with significant underlying cardiac pathology, it may be a normal variant in a minority of cases. Causes of LBBB include: cardio-myopathy, ischaemic heart disease (including acute MI), hypertension, aortic valve disease and right ventricular pacing. Clinical findings in subjects with LBBB will, to an extent, depend upon the exact nature of the underlying cardiac disease. For example, a displaced apex beat and third heart sound may be seen in dilated cardiomyopathy, while a fourth heart sound may be seen in cases of left ventricular hypertrophy or ischaemia. However, in all cases of LBBB there is early activation of the right side of the septum and the right ventricular myocardium. Trans-septal activation is trans-myocardial and hence slowed. This means that left ventricular activation and subsequent contraction is delayed in comparison to the right ventricle, resulting in the clinical finding of reversed splitting of the second heart sound. In this fit, asymptomatic man this is therefore likely to be the most frequently found physical sign.

.45   A: Acute rheumatic fever

Although the incidence of acute rheumatic fever has significantly declined in the western world, it is still a leading cause of cardiac morbidity in less industrialised countries. It occurs following infection with group A streptococ-cal species and it is thought that antigenic mimicry results in an autoimmune response and the subsequent clinical manifestations. The diagnosis is made clinically and generally involves the Jones criteria. To make the diagnosis there must be evidence of preceding streptococcal infection and either two major or one major and two minor criteria. In this case the patient has two major criteria – polyarthritis and evidence of carditis (most commonly involving the mitral valve, manifest as mitral incompetence). Other major criteria are chorea, erythema marginatum and subcutaneous nodules. This patient also has two minor criteria – fever and elevated inflammatory markers. Although SBE is a significant possibility the history is usually more prolonged. The mean age of presentation for atrial myxoma is in the fifth decade, although they have been described in younger subjects. Kawasaki disease (mucocutaneous lymph node syndrome) is a generalised vasculitis of unknown aetiology, with 80% of cases occurring in children under five years. Cardiac findings include pancarditis and coronary artery abnormalities. Systemic lupus erythematosus can have cardiac involvement (including pericarditis, myocarditis and, rarely, endocardi-tis) but the C-reactive protein (CRP) is not normally elevated.

1.46   B: Amiodarone and warfarin

Although this patient has lone AF (no obvious aetiology and normal cardiac structure) it is important to continue formal anticoagulation with warfarin for a period of at least 4 weeks after successful cardioversion. Atrial mechanical stunning occurs postcardioversion and lasts for several days and therefore patients remain at risk of thromboembolism even if atrial thrombi are excluded by preprocedural trans-oesophageal echocardiogram. Indeed, patients appear to be at particular risk when synchronised atrial contraction subsequently returns. In the peri-procedural period, amiodarone has been shown to help maintain sinus rhythm, at least in the short term, and most would agree to continue it until out-patient review.

1.47   B: Implantable cardioverter defibrillator

Following failed sudden cardiac death, in the absence of a reversible cause (e.g. acute myocardial infarction), current recommendations (*NICE Guidelines*) favour the insertion of an implantable cardioverter defibrillator (ICD). ICDs are indicated for spontaneous, sustained VT causing syncope or significant haemo-dynamic compromise or sustained VT in the setting of impaired left ventricular function (ejection fraction < 35%) and prior myocardial infarction. These patients are routinely treated with β-blockers. Those that experience shocks despite β-blockers need interrogation of the device, as it may be possible to program extra anti-tachycardia pacing. An additional anti-arrhythmic such as amiodarone may be prescribed, but beware that these increase the defibrilla-tion threshold.

1.48   B: Left internal mammary artery

The LAD supplies a major part of the left ventricular myocardium, including the anterior wall, apex and septum and as such it is important to choose the best option for revascularisation. The left internal mammary artery (LIMA) is usually free of atheroma and rarely develops intimal hyperplasia, unlike vein grafts. In contrast to the 40–60% patency seen in vein grafts at 10–12 years post-CABG, LIMA graft patency exceeds 90%. Patency for in-situ LIMA grafts appears better than free grafts. Therefore the origin of the LIMA from the left subclavian artery is normally left intact, while the distal vessel is carefully mobilised and eventually anastomosed to the LAD (pedicle LIMA graft).

1.49   B: Hypertrophic cardiomyopathy

The classic finding in hypertrophic cardiomyopathy (HCM) is inappropriate hypertrophy of the myocardium without obvious cause. The ventricular cavity

Answers: Cardiology

is usually small and microscopic examination reveals gross disorganisation of muscle bundles and myofibrillar disarray. Familial HCM is inherited in an autosomal dominant manner, accounting for approximately 50% of cases. It is thought that many of the sporadic cases result from spontaneous mutations. Although many patients are asymptomatic and identified by screening, symptoms include dyspnoea, classic angina, palpitations and dizziness. The majority of symptoms are exacerbated with exercise. There is a small risk of sudden cardiac death. Syncope may result from inadequate cardiac output during exercise or arrhythmias. The resting electrocardiogram (ECG) is usually abnormal and the commonest features include ST segment and T-wave abnormalities, LVH with the tallest complexes in the mid-precordial leads and prominent Q-waves (inferior and precordial). Left ventricular hypertrophy also occurs secondary to hypertension, aortic stenosis and due to Fabry's disease (a storage disorder involving the α-galactosidase enzyme). Supra-valvular aortic stenosis is seen in several different clinical settings, for example as a sporadic, isolated congenital lesion or as part of a clinical syndrome eg Williams' syndrome (elfin facies, mental impairment, hypercalcaemia and peripheral pulmonary stenoses).

.50   B: Endocardial cushion defect

The most common causes of morbidity and mortality in Down's syndrome are congenital heart defects, which are present in 40–50% of cases. The most characteristic cardiac abnormality is a defect of endocardial cushion closure. This results from varying degrees of incomplete development of the inferior portion of the atrial septum, the inflow portion of the ventricular septum and the atrioventricular valves. Therefore abnormalities may range from a small ostium primum ASD to an extensive defect that also involves the ventricular septum, together with the mitral and tricuspid valves. Patients with trisomy 21 seem to have a particular propensity to develop pulmonary hypertension in situations resulting in increased pulmonary blood flow, irrespective of the complexity of the underlying defect. Aortic and pulmonary valve cusps are predisposed to develop fenestrations in adulthood, resulting in valvular incompetence. Mitral valve prolapse is also found with increased frequency in Down's syndrome.

ANSWERS

Haematology

.1   **C: Serum lactate dehydrogenase (LDH) level of 1500 (normal 100–300 IU/l)**

An elevated reticulocyte count may be found in this situation as a result of recovery from blood loss associated with the Caesarean section. Increased megakaryocytes merely imply peripheral platelet destruction as the cause of the thrombocytopenia, examples being immune thrombocytopenia, disseminated intravascular coagulation (DIC), thrombotic thrombocytopenic purpura (TTP), haemolytic–uraemic syndrome (HUS) and hypersplenism. Gross elevation of LDH implies intravascular red cell destruction (by fibrin strands), an invariable accompaniment of TTP. Fragmented red cells may also be seen on the blood film. In TTP, the consumed coagulation factors (but not platelets) are replaced quickly enough to maintain relatively normal coagulation tests. In contrast, in DIC the coagulation factors are used up more quickly than they can be replaced, resulting in abnormal coagulation tests. Blood transfusion or pregnancy frequently results in the stimulation of the immune system to produce HLA antibodies, not related in any way to TTP.

.2   **C: Plasma exchange for fresh-frozen plasma**

The clinical scenario described is that of thrombotic thrombocytopenic purpura (TTP). In this situation, it is likely to be associated with ciclosporine therapy, which should be stopped. Other associations with TTP are quinine therapy, pregnancy and the puerperium, autoimmune disease and malignancy. Many cases are idiopathic. There is often an increased amount of high molecular weight 'sticky' von Willebrand factor (vWF) in the blood of TTP patients, which glues the platelets to the vascular endothelium, causing thrombocytopenia and micro-vascular occlusion. Platelet activation leads to the laying down of fibrin strands, which damage passing red blood cells causing microangiopathic haemolytic anaemia. In many cases, this sticky vWF is present because of the absence of a vWF-cleaving enzyme, ADAMST13, that normally splits high-molecular-weight into low-molecular-weight vWF. High volume daily plasma exchange replaces the vWF-cleaving protease and removes the high-molecular-weight vWF.

.3   **C: Autoimmune haemolytic anaemia**

She has a macrocytic anaemia with raised MCV. The absence of symptoms associated with a flare-up in her systemic lupus erythematosus (SLE) and an erythrocyte sedimentation rate (ESR) of only 24 (slightly raised because of the anaemia) imply that anaemia of chronic disease is not likely to be responsible and in any case is usually a normocytic anaemia. Iron deficiency causes a microcytic anaemia, as does thalassaemia trait. Both hypothyroidism and warm auto-immune haemolysis are associated with a macrocytic anaemia but only haemolysis is associates with an increased reticulocyte count. There is an association between immune haemolysis and thrombocytopenia and SLE.

2.4   C: Dry tap aspirate with increased reticulin on trephine biopsy

This man has a leucoerythroblastic anaemia, defined as the presence of nucleated red cells and primitive white cells of any variety in the peripheral blood. The causes of a leucoerythroblastic blood picture are either a very sick patient (trauma, operation, septicaemia, metabolic upset) obviously not present here or marrow infiltration. While secondary deposits in marrow from carcinoma of prostate, breast, lung, thyroid or kidney can cause leucoerythroblastic anaemia, they do not generally cause hepatosplenomegaly. The finding of marrow cells in the liver biopsy is termed extramedullary haemopoiesis and is diagnostic of a myeloproliferative disorder. The four myeloproliferative disorders are primary polycythaemia, primary thrombocythaemia, myelofibrosis and chronic myeloid leukaemia. Myelofibrosis is usually associated with leucoerythroblastic anaemia, with tear-drop poikilocytes in the blood, dry tap marrow aspirate and increased reticulin and fibrosis on marrow trephine biopsy. The white cell count and platelet count may be low, normal or high and the spleen is often palpably enlarged.

2.5   E: Continue warfarin at same dose

A previous DVT predisposes to further DVTs so there is probably not enough evidence to embark on a thrombophilia screen in this case. Both protein C and protein S are natural anticoagulants that are vitamin K dependent so screening for their deficiency when established on warfarin is very difficult as levels may be reduced by coumarin therapy. Similarly, heparin therapy may reduce antithrombin levels. It is usually best to continue anticoagulation for the usual period and then stop it, performing thrombophilia screen after at least a month off. Low-dose aspirin therapy will not interfere. Activated protein C resistance testing (APCR) is a screening test for factor V Leiden. It detects the lack of prolongation of a clotting test when protein C is added to a patient's plasma the activated factor V in the plasma cannot be inactivated by the protein C. Such a failure of neutralisation may be found when the factor V has genetically abnormal structure such a factor V Leiden. The abnormality may be confirmed by PCR screening tests. An INR range of 2–3 is usually aimed for in warfarin anticoagulation after DVT.

Answers: Haematology

2.6   A: Irradiated fully crossmatched red cells

Irradiation is used to kill the lymphocytes that may cause third-party graft versus host disease. This is due to immuno-competent lymphocytes in the transfused cellular blood product settling in an immuno-compromised recipient, proliferating and fighting the recipient's tissues. Patients who are considered immunodeficient enough to require irradiated blood products are Hodgkin disease, severe combined congenital immunodeficiency, post-organ transplant (or less that one month pre-organ transplant) and patients who have been treated with nucleoside analogues such as fludarabine. Since this patient has already been infected with, and therefore will carry, the cytomegalovirus (CMV) virus he does not require CMV-negative blood. His anaemia is relatively chronic and he is haemodynamically stable so abbreviated or uncrossmatched blood is not required. Whole blood is no longer available.

2.7   C: Tear drops

The patient has the classical findings of myelofibrosis and tear-drop poikilocytes would be expected in the blood. Burr cells (shaped like the burr seeds that catch on clothing) are found in chronic renal failure. Helmet cells are half red cells that have been chopped in half by a fibrin strand in micro-angiopathic haemolytic states. Red cell cytoskeleton abnormalities, such as hereditary elliptocytosis or spherocytosis, may cause congenital haemolytic anaemias. Pencil cells are long thin red cells that accompany microcytosis and hypochromia in iron deficiency anaemia. Sickle cells should be obvious!

2.8   E: Sickle cell disease

Pernicious anaemia is found with increasing frequency the more north the latitude, though no race is exempt from this auto-immune disease. Beta-thalassaemia is associated with a congenital inability to make the β chains of adult haemoglobin. The word thalassic is derived from the Greek for 'the sea' since most of the original cases were found around the Mediterranean. Alpha-thalassaemia is more common in patients of Chinese or Far Eastern origin. Glucose-6-phosphate dehydrogenase (G6PD) deficiency is a sex-linked disorder associated with paroxysmal haemolysis in response to oxidant stress induced by drugs, foodstuffs (favism) and infection. Leishmaniasis is a parasitic infection spread by the sandfly and found in Greece, Spain and other Mediterranean countries with increasing frequency. Global warming may cause northern spread. Although sickle cell disease is classically found in sub-Saharan Africa it is widely disseminated.

2.9   D: Disseminated intravascular coagulation

Idiopathic thrombocytopenia (ITP), TTP and HUS are all associated with increased platelet destruction. In ITP the platelets are destroyed in the reticulo-endothelial system as the result of an immune mediated destruction. In TTP and HUS the platelets become glued to the inside of the blood vessels; here they become activated, triggering coagulation and the laying down of fibrin strands. These strands damage passing red blood cells causing a micro-angiopathic haemolytic anaemia. However the coagulation factors are consumed relatively slowly and hence abnormality of the coagulation screening tests or clinical bleeding in TTP and HUS is relatively unusual. In DIC activation of the coagulation system, usually by release into the circulation of a pro-coagulant, consumes all clotting factors and platelets. Bleeding in DIC is compounded by hyperfibrinolysis. The May–Hegglin anomaly is an autosomally dominant inherited congenital thrombocytopenia associated with large platelets in the blood and cytoplasmic inclusions (Döhle bodies) in the granulocytes.

2.10   D: Patchy PET-FDG active lesions in lumbar and thoracic vertebrae

In MGUS there will not usually be impairment of renal function, lytic lesions or hypercalcaemia. The paraprotein is of low level (<10 g/l if IgG) and does not increase significantly over time. About 1% of MGUS turn into myeloma for each year of follow-up. The number of plasma cells found in the bone marrow in myeloma is subject to sampling error – if the aspiration needle hits a lytic lesion then this can be 100%, if it samples a relatively normal area of marrow it can be normal – less than 5%. PET-FDG scans are rarely required in myeloma management but if done will highlight myeloma deposits. About 20% of MGUS patients may have reduction in one or more of the non-paraprotein immunoglobulins. Essentially the diagnosis of MGUS is made by excluding a diagnosis of myeloma.

2.11   B: Plasma viscosity

The clinical picture in this case is that of Waldenstrom's macroglobulinaemia. The blood and clinical picture is very similar to chronic lymphocytic leukaemia (CLL) with lymphocytosis and lymphadenopathy and hepatosplenomegaly. The lymphocytes are often intermediate in morphology between small lymphocytes of CLL and plasma cells of myeloma. An IgM paraprotein is produced. Because of the large molecular size of the IgM molecules plasma hyperviscosity may be seen even at relatively low paraprotein concentrations. Normal plasma viscosity is in the range of 1.4–2.0 mPa but is usually over 4.0 in plasma hyperviscosity syndrome. In this condition bleeding (due to impaired platelet function in

Answers: Haematology

the sticky plasma), oedema and cerebral and renal dysfunction are commonly seen. The presence of a paraprotein is suggested by the very high ESR in the presence of a relatively low CRP.

2.12   D: Reduced plasma haptoglobin

The body tries to prevent free haemoglobin in the plasma disappearing into the urine and it is initially bound to haptoglobin that then returns to the liver, so reduced haptoglobin levels are a sensitive test for intravascular haemolysis. Haemoglobin in plasma then binds to albumin, which may be detected by the Schumm's test for methaemalbumin. Free haemoglobin will then pass into the glomerular filtrate. Even here some haemoglobin is taken up by the tubular lining cells and converted to haemosiderin. These cells are later shed into the urine and can be detected by a positive urinary haemosiderin – a way of picking up an episode of intravascular haemolysis that has passed. It will take days for a reticulocyte response to anaemia to develop and for erythroid hyperplasia to generate more red cells.

2.13   E: Spectroscopic examination of haemoglobin

Cyanosis in the absence of hypoxia may be due to methaemoglobinaemia. Haemoglobin becomes oxidised to the ferric form and this has a browny colour when seen in the blood sample tube and results in a bluish discoloration impossible to distinguish from cyanosis. Methaemoglobinaemia may be due to an abnormal haemoglobin – haemoglobin M or a defect in the enzyme systems usually responsible for reducing small amounts of methaemoglobin that are continuously formed to normal haemoglobin. This is most commonly methaemoglobin reductase deficiency. Mildly affected individuals may be normal but develop symptoms when challenged with drugs such as dapsone, nitrates (eg GTN, nitrate contamination of drinking water) or aniline dyes. Babies may be particularly susceptible. This patient had recently started dapsone treatment for her skin condition. Spectroscopy of haemoglobin will allow identification of the methaemoglobin and treatment may be given with intravenous methylene blue.

2.14   E: Prescription of simvastatin 2 weeks ago has caused warfarin over-anticoagulation

Increased alcohol consumption (eg the unexpected party) results in over-anticoagulation, not reduction in regular intake. A regular life-style makes for good warfarin control. Warfarin reduces coagulation factor II, VII, IX and X. With the exception of factor VII, deficiencies of these factors IX will prolong the APTT, particularly if over-anticoagulated. Modest increase in D-dimers may be found in cases of thrombosis and haematoma, allowing D-dimer to be used as part of a diagnostic algorithm in suspected DVT. Green vegetables such as spinach, kale and sprouts are rich in vitamin K and antagonise warfarin effect. The INR is usually checked for normality at the start of warfarin treatment. Drugs that commonly cause increased warfarin effect are broad-spectrum antibiotics, selective serotonin re-uptake inhibitors (SSRIs), azoles, anabolic steroids, statins and amiodarone. Check *Interactions Appendix* in *BNF* and check INR a few days after starting a new drug.

2.15   D: Primary polycythaemia rubra vera

This young woman presents with the classic findings of Budd–Chiari syndrome, which may sometimes be seen in patients taking the oestrogen-containing oral contraceptive pill (OCP), but nevertheless a thrombophilia screen is indicated, fortunately performed before starting anticoagulation which makes the results of such investigations very difficult to interpret. Although the microcytosis, hypochromia and low serum ferritin confirm iron deficiency, she is not anaemic. Prescription of OCP reveals her polycythaemia, previously held in check by iron deficiency. Iron deficiency is common in primary polycythaemia because a large amount of iron is required to make a big red cell mass, venesection is the most popular method of treatment and the platelet function deficiency found in all the myeloproliferative disorders may contribute to occult bleeding. The presence of neutrophilia and thrombocytosis help confirm primary rather than secondary polycythaemia as the diagnosis and this may be confirmed by looking for the JAK2 mutation present in 90% of cases of primary polycythaemia.

2.16   D: It contains all the coagulation factors, albumin and immunoglobulin

The optimum replacement fluid after major burns is albumin as large amounts of this weep from denuded body surfaces. Albumin, unlike FFP, is heat treated to inactivate viruses and does not contain blood group antibodies. Fresh-frozen plasma is commonly used for the replacement of multiple coagulation factor deficiencies such as those found in disseminated intravascular coagulation, warfarin overdose with haemorrhage and after massive stored blood transfusion. FFP contains blood group antibodies and therefore the patient's blood group should be known. If not, group AB fresh-frozen plasma does not contain anti-A or anti-B antibodies, so can be given to recipients of any ABO blood group. FFP takes 30–40 minutes to thaw in a 37 °C water-bath so is not immediately available for administration.

Answers: Haematology

2.17   C: Idiopathic cold haemagglutinin disease

This woman has cold agglutinins and low-grade B-cell lymphoproliferative disorders, and infection with Epstein-Barr virus (EBV) or *Mycoplasma pneumoniae* are potential causes. She does not have a lymphocytosis, which would be expected in CLL, and physical examination would be expected to show evidence of active infection. Glandular fever is unusual in the elderly. This leaves idiopathic cold haemagglutinin disease as the most likely diagnosis. Many of these cases eventually turn out to have an underlying low-grade B-cell lymphoma if careful clonality studies are done on the bone marrow lymphocytes. Unlike warm auto-immune haemolytic anaemia, which is usually steroid-responsive, in cold agglutinin disease the act of keeping warm or chlorambucil or rituximab use are the most effective treatments. Tertiary syphilis is historically associated with paroxysmal cold haemoglobinuria (PCH), in which a cold-acting IgG antibody causes intravascular haemolysis by activating complement rather than by causing red cell agglutination. Cold agglutinins are IgM antibodies. In modern times PCH is most commonly seen in children with viral infections.

2.18   E: Von Willebrand disease

The platelet count is normal and the only abnormality of coagulation screening is a slightly prolonged APTT. The PFA-100 test or 'in-vitro bleeding time' tests the ability of the patient's platelets to form a platelet haemostatic plug (closure time) in response to adrenaline and ADP. Aspirin will prolong the adrenaline-induced closure time, but will not prolong the ADP induced closure time. If both are prolonged there is a defect of platelet function. In association with the slightly prolonged APTT and relevant family history this is most likely to be von Willebrand disease (vWD). Von Willebrand factor (vWF) has two important functions. It allows platelets to attach to vascular sub-endothelial tissues and hence patients with vWD suffer platelet-type bleeding with muco-cutaneous bruising, purpura, nosebleeds, menorrhagia and post-traumatic bleeding. Von Willebrand factor also acts a protective carrier for coagulation factor VIII. Without vWF, factor VIII, is more rapidly degraded and hence there may be prolongation of the APTT, but not to the extent found in haemophilia A.

2.19   B: Hodgkin's disease

Adenocarcinoma of lung is unlikely in this young non-smoking man and sufficient lymph node enlargement to cause vena caval obstruction is rare in sarcoidosis and tuberculosis. Seminoma would usually spread first to abdominal para-aortic lymph nodes. Weight loss, night sweats and fever are the 'B' symptoms found in lymphomas, which adversely affect prognosis. Alcohol-induced pain in the affected lymph nodes is a characteristic finding in Hodgkin's disease.

2.20   E: Hydroxycarbamide

This woman has a clear diagnosis of essential thrombocythaemia, with a platelet count over 1000×10^9/l and no evidence of an inflammatory, neoplastic or infective disease to cause a reactive thrombocytosis of this extent. Treatment should be directed at preventing further problems with platelet micro-vascular obstruction in the brain by platelet function inhibitors, such as aspirin or clopidogrel and reducing the platelet count to levels below 500×10^9/l by hydroxycarbamide (hydroxyurea) or anagrelide. There is no evidence of thrombosis or embolus so warfarin/heparin anticoagulation is not indicated. Iron deficiency has been correctly excluded as a driver to thrombocytosis in this case. Vincristine is a cytotoxic agent used in the lymphomas and lymphoblastic leukaemia and paradoxically may sometime increase the platelet count.

2.21   E: Induction chemotherapy would usually consist of cytosine and an anthracycline

Young patients with acute myeloid leukaemia (AML) are treated with conventional chemotherapy if the prognosis appears good and bone marrow transplant (associated with a higher treatment-related mortality) if the prognosis appears poor with conventional treatment. Cytogenetic abnormality and response to the first course of chemotherapy determine prognosis in AML. Three cytogenetic abnormalities that are associated with a good prognosis are: t(8;21) – commonest in the FAB morphological type M2; t(15;17) – found in acute promyelocytic leukaemia; and inversion 16 – found in acute myelomonocytic leukaemia with increased eosinophils. Three cytogenetic abnormalities that are associated with a particularly poor prognosis and recommendation to bone marrow allograft are: t(9;22) – the truncated chromosome 22 being the Philadelphia chromosome; and deletion of all or part of chromosomes 5 or 7. Failure to go into remission after the first course of treatment is also bad news. Vincristine and steroids are the principal remission-inducing drugs for acute lymphoblastic leukaemia, whereas cytosine and an anthracycline will almost always feature in an AML-induction regimen. A high-risk matched unrelated donor transplant is not justified in this young woman with good-prognosis cytogenetics unless she fails to go into remission with the first course of chemotherapy.

Answers: Haematology

2.22   A: The clinical and pathological features may all be related to the post-ictal state

This woman has a history typical of thrombotic thrombocytopenic purpura (TTP). An excess of high-molecular-weight von Willebrand's factor sticks platelets to the inside of her vascular endothelium, resulting in their activation and local triggering of the coagulation cascade. Fibrin formation in small blood vessels chops up passing red cells, resulting in anaemia and reticulocytosis. Some of these red cells can re-seal, continuing as half red cells (helmet cells) or, if subject to multiple fibrin collisions, as fragmented cells. Such a micro-angiopathic blood picture may be found in other conditions such as dissemi-nated intravascular coagulation, but in this condition abnormality of the coagulation screening tests would be expected. Infection with *E. coli* O157 may precipitate haemolytic–uraemic syndrome, in which renal failure is a major feature as opposed to neurological problems as in TTP.

2.23   B: Stainable bone marrow iron

There is a high probability of iron deficiency due to menorrhagia and a diet with inadequate red meat, which is the richest source of dietary iron. Serum ferritin is reduced in iron deficiency and increased in iron overload and provides a useful guide to body iron stores. However, it may be falsely elevated into the normal range in patients who have an inflammatory condition as ferritin is an acute phase reactant, similar to CRP, immunoglobulins and fibrinogen. In iron deficiency there will be no stainable iron in the bone marrow though this investigation is too invasive to perform in the diagnosis of most cases! It is possible to have a normal haemoglobin level but no stainable iron stores if iron from broken-down red cells is efficiently reprocessed into haemoglobin. In iron deficiency the serum iron is low and the total iron-binding capacity (TIBC – equivalent to transferrin) is raised. Dividing one by the other gives a reduced transferrin saturation in iron deficiency. Measurement of zinc protoporphyrin is used as a screening test for iron deficiency, when it is elevated. In β-thalassaemia trait, which would be in the differential diagnosis of this girl's microcytic anaemia, an elevated haemoglobin A_2 level is a common finding. Inability to make the β-globin chains of haemoglobin A results in compensation by making more haemoglobin A_2 which does not need β-globin chains, having instead δ-globin chains.

2.24   E: Diastolic murmur at the cardiac apex

In β-thalassaemia major virtually no chains can be manufactured and conse-quently progressive anaemia results during the attempted physiological switch from haemoglobin (Hb) F to Hb A during the first year of life. Nucleated red

Answers: Haematology

cells are a consistent feature of the blood film in β-thalassaemia major and help to differentiate this condition from other causes of severe microcytic anaemia such as iron deficiency. In the untransfused patient skeletal changes such as pushing forward of the mandible and maxilla (prognathism), bossing of skull and stunting of growth may be found. These skeletal changes are secondary to the severe erythroid hyperplasia, most of which is ineffective in maintaining a normal haemoglobin level. Regular blood transfusions are required as well as a chelating agent such as desferrioxamine to prevent iron overload that results in cardiomyopathy, endocrinopathy and cirrhosis. An ejection systolic murmur may be heard in any severe form of anaemia due to increased blood flow through the heart, but not a diastolic murmur.

2.25 C: Repeat coagulation screen on fresh sample

A prolonged thrombin time in isolation, in this clinical situation, is most likely to have resulted from heparin contamination of the blood sample used for the coagulation screen. It is likely to have been drawn from an indwelling catheter with insufficient removal of heparin-contaminated blood. A repeat coagulation screen on a fresh sample is likely to be normal. The thrombin time is not used for dose control of conventional heparin because it is so sensitive to heparin effect, the APTT being a better substitute. Sometimes it is possible for the laboratory to neutralise the heparin in the sample with protamine to demonstrate that the prolonged thrombin time is an artefact due to heparin contamination. Prolongation of the thrombin time may be seen in heparin, disseminated intravascular coagulation (DIC) and in the presence of a low fibrinogen. Measurement of FDPs is a reasonable option in DIC but these may be elevated in a trauma case.

2.26 B: Coagulation screen

This woman has a deep venous thrombosis and probable pulmonary embolus in the puerperal period. There is a clear clinical reason for the thrombosis and in the absence of a personal or family history of thrombosis, screening for thrombophilia is not indicated. There is no reason to measure clotting factor IX. A coagulation screen may reasonably be performed before starting patients on anticoagulant therapy as a baseline.

2.27 D: Continue heparin infusion at current rate

The aim of conventional heparin therapy, which should be given by continuous infusion to maintain constant blood levels, is to prolong the APTT by 1.5–2.5 times the control value. This woman is therefore adequately anticoagulated

Answers: Haematology

and she may continue conventional heparin treatment. The equivalence of low-molecular-weight heparin in the treatment of pulmonary embolism has been shown but it has not been demonstrated to be superior and is considerably more expensive. Warfarin treatment takes 72 hours to take full effect; therefore heparin treatment will need to be continued until the INR (measuring warfarin effect) exceeds 2.0.

2.28   E: Balanced expression of kappa and lambda light chain of surface immunoglobulin on blood lymphocytes

More than 95% of cases of chronic lymphocytic leukaemia are of B-cell lineage. Curiously, they almost always express a T-cell antigen CD5, as well as the usual B-cell antigens such as CD19. B cells are responsible for immunoglobulin production and there may be deranged antibody production, with low immunoglobulin levels associated with predisposition to infection and auto-immune phenomena of which the commonest is a positive direct antiglobulin test, sometimes associated with warm auto-immune haemolytic anaemia. Establishment of clonality is important in the diagnosis of neoplasia and one would expect these lymphocytes to all express kappa light chains or all express lambda. Balanced production would be more in keeping with a reactive lymphocytosis, but if the other investigations suggest CLL this test should probably be repeated.

2.29   D: Multiple myeloma

It is quite reasonable to investigate this girl for any of the first three causes of macrocytosis. Folate deficiency may be caused by antiepileptic medication and it is controversial whether the fits get worse if the folate deficiency is corrected. Liver disease causes macrocytosis by interfering with the construction of the lipid bilayer of the red cell membrane. The occurrence of multiple myeloma would be exceptional in a girl of this age group, though macrocytosis is found in patients with multiple myeloma. There is no particular reason why she should have auto-immune haemolytic anaemia and this is fairly low down the list of diagnostic possibilities.

2.30   C: Factor VIII inhibitor screen

The most likely cause of his persistent haemarthrosis is the development of antibodies against factor VIII, although many haemophiliacs do develop a 'target joint' subject to recurrent haemarthrosis due to synovial hyperplasia and secondary joint damage. This is a difficult situation to treat. The most relevant investigation to detect these would be a screen for factor VIII inhibitor antibodies. He is unlikely to have developed gout. Joint aspiration is rarely performed in haemophilia, effective correction of the coagulation abnormality being the best treatment.

2.31   E: Measurement of CD55 and CD59 surface antigen on peripheral blood leucocytes and platelets

The history is typical of paroxysmal nocturnal haemoglobinuria (PNH). In this rare disorder there is complement-mediated lysis of red cells, white cells and platelets, resulting in a pancytopenia. Sometimes haematopoietic stem cells are also affected, giving rise to aplastic anaemia. Intravascular lysis of red cells results in haemoglobinuria and the release of tissue factor from lysed cells gives an acquired thrombophilia, so that patients may present with thrombotic problems that are a common cause of death in this disease. The disease is due to the lack of a transmembrane glycoprotein that acts as an anchor for various molecules, including complement activators and CD antigens. Although Ham' test is usually positive in PNH, in this case the patient has been transfused with normal red cells so this may result in a negative result as red cells are used for this test. The membrane defect can however be revealed by measurement of antigens such as CD55 and CD59 on other blood cells. Urinary haemosiderin merely tells us that the patient has had chronic haemoglobinuria, some of the haemoglobin being internalised within tubular cells, which are later shed into the urinary deposit and give a positive stain for iron. The Donath–Landsteiner test detects the complement-dependent, cold-acting antibody found in paroxysmal cold haemoglobinuria, a different disease.

2.32   C: It is free of risk of hepatitis transmission

Cryoprecipitate is prepared by thawing fresh-frozen plasma, when curd-like precipitate forms at the bottom of the bag that may be harvested and is particularly rich in fibrinogen factor VII and von Willebrand's factor. Because heat-detergent inactivates concentrates of factor VII and von Willebrand's factor these are preferred for the treatment of von Willebrand's disease rather than cryoprecipitate, which has not gone through a viral inactivation stage and therefore may carry a very small risk of hepatitis transmission. Cryoprecipitate is most commonly used for the correction of a low fibrinogen in patients with disseminated intravascular coagulation or massive transfusion. The von Willebrand's factor in the cryoprecipitate can ameliorate bleeding in uraemic patients but desmopressin (DDAVP) administration causes endothelial cells to secrete stored von Willebrand's factor and may be a more suitable treatment of uraemic platelet defect.

Answers: Haematology

2.33   D: G-CSF carries no risk of viral transmission

G-CSF is a recombinant protein and therefore there is no risk of viral disease transmission. G-CSF stimulates committed myeloid progenitor cells and is therefore of most use when the primitive stem cells have differentiated into the early myeloid lineage. It may shorten periods of post-chemotherapy neutropenia by a few days. It is best given after chemotherapy rather than immediately before as it may stimulate granulocyte precursors into division, making them more susceptible to the suppressive effects of cytotoxic chemotherapy. Most modern trials have shown the benefits of accelerated chemotherapy rather than increasing the interval between courses to allow full count recovery.

2.34   B: Recent febrile illness associated with high titres against parvovirus B19

Chemotherapy and radiotherapy are the most common causes of a hypoplastic marrow with pancytopenia. Busulfan is an old-fashioned cytotoxic treatment for CML, but is still used and the possibility of deliberate poisoning should always be considered. An idiosyncratic reaction to drugs may result in aplastic anaemia; phenylbutazone and chloramphenicol are well-known examples. If in doubt the drug should be stopped or changed. A severe aplastic anaemia can follow any viral hepatitis, often after recovery of the liver function tests. PNH has an association with aplastic anaemia, as the haematopoietic stem cells are more liable to complement lysis, like the cells in the peripheral blood. Parvovirus B19 causes pure red cell aplasia, not aplastic anaemia. It infects the erythroblasts in the bone marrow, shutting down red cell production for a few days. In normal people, whose red cells have a 3-month lifespan, stopping red cell production for a few days is of no consequence, but in patients with chronic congenital haemolytic anaemia a severe anaemia may result in aplastic crisis. However the white cell and platelet counts remain normal and this is not true of aplastic anaemia.

2.35   C: The patient is unusually sensitive to the effect of warfarin

The heparin dose should be adjusted to obtain an APTT ratio of 1.5 to 2.5. This patient is correctly heparinised. Over-heparinisation can cause prolongation of the INR, which normally reflects warfarin effect. Achieving an INR of 1.8 only 12 hours after the first dose indicates increased warfarin sensitivity or abnormal liver function tests at the start of therapy; normally the effects of warfarin are not seen for 48–72 hours after starting treatment. The therapeutic INR range for DVT/PE and AF is 2–3; for recurrent thrombosis on warfarin or artificial heart valves the range is 3–4.5. The INR is the prothrombin ratio raised to the power of the sensitivity index of the thromboplastin used in the test. In simpler terms it is the prothrombin ratio multiplied by a 'fiddle factor' to bring it in line with the results of other laboratories, so that the INR should be the same in any laboratory performing the test.

2.36   E: Elevated TSH and low free thyroxine

Beta-thalassaemia trait results in a microcytic hypochromic anaemia difficult to differentiate from iron deficiency except that the haemoglobin is usually over 9 g/dl. Consequently, this woman is much more likely to have iron deficiency. In pernicious anaemia lack of gastric acid prevents iron being split from protein to allow its absorption, so patients with this disease frequently suffer iron deficiency. Non-steroidal anti-inflammatory drug (NSAID) treatment may cause gastric erosions and impair platelet function, enhancing chronic gastrointestinal (GI) bleeding that may result in iron deficiency. The most easily absorbed form of iron in the diet is in red meat and vegetarians have a more precarious iron status than meat eaters. The anaemia of hypothyroidism is usually macrocytic rather than microcytic.

2.37   D: Anorexia and malaise

Increase in haemoglobin level results in an increased whole blood viscosity that may exacerbate hypertension already present in patients with renal failure. Increased blood viscosity may also predispose to a higher incidence of thrombosis and it is usual to limit the haemoglobin level to around 10 g/dl in renal patients. Improvement in haemoglobin level often results in a greater feeling elling of wellbeing and improved appetite. Pure red cell aplasia is a very rare unwanted effect of erythropoietin administration due to the stimulation of antibodies by administered EPO that crossreacts with the patient's endogenous erythropoietin. A similar problem has been reported in trials of human recombinant thrombopoietin.

2.38   B: Haemoglobin electrophoresis

This man has leucoerythroblastic anaemia: nucleated red cells and primitive white cells in the peripheral blood. Unless the patient is seriously ill this is likely to be due to bone marrow infiltration. Investigations should include a search for primary tumours that characteristically metastasise to bone (lung, thyroid, kidney, breast, and prostate) as well as haematological malignancies such as myeloma.

2.39   C: The ABO type of individuals can change during some illnesses, eg acute myeloid leukaemia

Naturally occurring anti-A and anti-B antibodies are IgM (agglutinating and nonplacental-passing). IgG antibodies may be made in response to immunological stimulation by incompatible red cells such as those transmitted from fetus to mother during pregnancy. These IgG anti-A or anti-B antibodies may cause ABO haemolytic disease of the newborn. Changing of an ABO blood group is an exceptional event but may be found after bone marrow transplantation, in some cases of acute myeloid leukaemia affecting the erythroid lineage and in some cases of enteric disease when the red cells of non-group B individuals may acquire a B antigen. Group O is the commonest blood group in all races. People who are group O are universal donors for red cells but people of blood group AB are universal donors for fresh-frozen plasma as their plasma contains neither anti-A nor anti-B.

2.40   A: Stop heparin and commence heparinoid

The history is strongly suggestive of heparin-induced thrombocytopenia (HIT). This condition is associated with immunological activation of platelets and an increased risk of further thrombosis. Anticoagulation should not be stopped. HIT may be seen with low molecular weight heparin so this is not a suitable alternative. Either a heparinoid such as danaparoid or recombinant hirudin should be used, after taking haematological advice.

2.41   E: Thrombotic thrombocytopenic purpura

Thrombotic thrombocytopenic purpura is a disorder characterised by severe thrombocytopenia, purpura, fragmentation haemolysis and ischaemic organ damage to the brain and kidney. Extensive deposition of arterial thrombi occurs. An immune-mediated mechanism involving the production of an antibody, which inhibits von Willebrand's factor (cleaving protease), has been described. Plasma exchange and plasma infusions are the most effective therapy. Aspirin, corticosteroids and other agents, such as vincristine, azathioprine and cyclophosphamide may be of benefit. Haemolytic–uraemic syndrome in children is a similar disorder but damage is confined to the kidney.

2.42   A: Major ABO incompatibility

Haemolytic transfusion reactions can be immediate or delayed. Immediate life threatening reactions with massive intravascular haemolysis are caused by complement-activating IgG or IgM antibodies. These are usually ABO anti-

Answers: Haematology

bodies and the severity depends on the recipient's titre of antibody. Reactions can occur after the transfusion of only a few millilitres of blood. Immediate clinical features include back pain, flushing, headache, shortness of breath, vomiting, rigors, urticaria, pyrexia, tachycardia and hypotension. Many of these features will be masked in the anaesthetised patient. Evidence of red cell destruction with haemoglobinuria and disseminated intravascular coagulation can occur. In the UK all such incidents are reported through the SHOT (serious hazards of transfusion) system and they should be investigated locally.

2.43   D: Hereditary spherocytosis

Hereditary spherocytosis is the commonest hereditary haemolytic anaemia in Northern Europeans. Inheritance is usually autosomal dominant but can be autosomal recessive. It is due to a defect in the structural proteins of the red cell membrane, including ankyrin, anion exchanger, protein 4.2 and spectrin. The patients present with anaemia, fluctuating jaundice, splenomegaly and pigment gallstones. The degree of anaemia tends to be the same in families. The blood film shows microspherocytes. Patients' red cells show increased haemolysis compared to normal in the osmotic fragility test. The mainstay of treatment is splenectomy in those who have sufficient haemolysis to justify this or gallstones.

2.44   B: Chronic myeloid leukaemia

Chronic myeloid leukaemia is an acquired clonal proliferative disorder. In most cases there is a reciprocal translocation between the long arms of chromosomes 9 and 22 resulting in an abnormal chromosome 22 (the Philadelphia chromosome) and the formation of a new fusion gene, *bcr/abl*. Clinically, the patients are often middle-aged but can present in any age group. Symptoms are related to anaemia and the raised white cell count. There is usually splenomegaly, which may be symptomatic. The white cell count is raised up to 500 × 10^9/l with a complete spectrum of cells in the peripheral blood, anaemia and often a raised platelet count. Agents like hydroxyurea and busulfan control the white cell count. Allogeneic bone marrow transplant offers the chance of cure in suitable candidates. The new tyrosine kinase inhibitor, STI 571 (Glivec) may be an important agent in the treatment of the disease. The natural course of the disease involves transformation to acute leukaemia in a median period of 3 to 4 years.

Answers: Haematology

2.45   C: Multiple myeloma

Multiple myeloma is characterised by a neoplastic monoclonal proliferation of plasma cells in the bone marrow. Clinical features include bone pain and pathological fractures, anaemia, recurrent infections, abnormal bleeding tendency, renal failure and hyperviscosity syndrome. It is diagnosed by finding two out of three of: (1) a paraprotein band in the serum or urine or both; (2) increased and often abnormal plasma cells in the bone marrow; and (3) lytic lesions on skeletal survey. Treatment involves resuscitation, treatment of renal failure, pain relief and, in older patients, melphalan and prednisolone. In younger patients more intensive combination chemotherapy regimens and a bone marrow transplant procedure may be considered.

2.46   B: Vitamin B$_{12}$, folic acid and iron supplements and slow transfusion of 1–2 units of packed cells if clinically indicated

Addisonian pernicious anaemia due to vitamin B$_{12}$ deficiency is usually caused by atrophy of the stomach, which is probably autoimmune in origin. It is more common in women than in men and the peak incidence is in older age groups. Patients present insidiously with gradual onset of symptoms and signs of anaemia and mild jaundice due to increased haemoglobin breakdown. Treatment with vitamin B$_{12}$ and folic acid is usually given until the exact vitamin deficiency is determined and also oral iron as requirements can increase when red cell production commences. Potassium levels should be monitored and potassium replacement may be required. Heart failure should be corrected. Blood transfusion should be avoided as it may cause circulatory overload. If judged to be essential because of anoxia, however, 1–2 units should be given slowly with the possibility of exchange transfusion being considered.

2.47   C: Glucose-6-phosphate dehydrogenase (G6PD) deficiency

Glucose-6-phosphate dehydrogenase oxidises glucose-6-phosphate (G6P) to 6- phosphogluconolactone (6PG) with concomitant reduction of nicotinamide adenine dinucleotide phosphate (NADP) to the reduced form NADPH. G6PD is essential to protect red cells from oxidative damage. The gene is located on the long arm of the X chromosome (Xq28). The deficiency affects over 400 million people world-wide. In most cases it exists as a balanced polymorphism, affected individuals having the advantage of resistance to malaria. Most people are asymptomatic unless exposed to an oxidising agent but a small subset of cases have chronic haemolysis. On exposure to infection or drugs or on ingestion of fava beans, patients rapidly develop intravascular haemolysis with haemoglobinuria. The blood film shows 'bite' cells and 'blister' cells, which have had Heinz bodies (oxidised denatured haemoglobin) removed by the spleen. Treatment consists of stopping the offending drug, maintaining a high urine output and transfusing if necessary.

2.48   E: Sideroblastic anaemia

In sideroblastic anaemia there are hypochromic red cells in the peripheral blood (suggesting iron deficiency) but increased bone marrow iron. Erythroblasts contain abnormal iron granules, characteristically in the mitochondria positioned round the nucleus, hence they are known as ring sideroblasts. There is a defect of haem synthesis. It is classified into hereditary and acquired forms. The hereditary form may be due to α-aminolevulinate synthase-2 deficiency. Acquired forms include myelodysplasia, drugs, including antituberculous medication and alcohol. Some patients may respond to pyridoxine and folic acid but blood transfusion may be the only way to maintain the haemoglobin.

2.49   A: Immediate exchange transfusion

Sickle cell anaemia may remain undiagnosed until adult life and a crisis can be precipitated by a move to a colder climate. Prophylactic treatment includes avoidance of factors likely to cause crisis, good general nutrition, folic acid, pneumococcal vaccination and oral penicillin. Crises are treated with rehydration, antibiotics if infection is a factor and strong analgesics. Exchange transfusion is indicated if there is neurological damage, visceral sequestration crises or recurrent painful crises. Achieving a haemoglobin (Hb) S level of less than 30% may limit the neurological damage. There may be problems in obtaining compatible blood for transfusion.

2.50   E: Beta-thalassaemia major

Beta-thalassaemia is usually due to deletions of the α-globin gene. There are two β-globin genes on each chromosome 16. All four genes must be deleted for β-thalassaemia major to occur. In some populations with β-thalassaemia trait one β-globin gene is missing on each chromosome 16 and so full-blown β-thalassaemia will not occur in offspring of affected parents. However, in other ethnic groups such as Chinese populations, individuals with β-thalassaemia trait tend to have two missing β-globin genes on the same chromosome 16 and so if both parents have the trait there is a one in four chance that the fetus will have β-thalassaemia major, which leads to failure of fetal haemoglobin production and death in-utero from hydrops fetalis.

Answers: Haematology

ANSWERS

Respiratory Medicine

RESPIRATORY MEDICINE: 'BEST OF FIVE' ANSWERS

.1   **D: Lupus pernio**

According to the American Thoracic Society (ATS) statement on sarcoidosis, the following are adverse prognostic factors for sarcoidosis:

- age of onset > 40 years old
- Afro-Caribbean or African-American race
- cardiac involvement
- chronic hypercalcaemia
- nephrocalcinosis
- chronic uveitis
- cystic bone lesions
- lupus pernio
- nasal mucosal involvement
- neurosarcoidosis
- progressive pulmonary sarcoidosis.

Smoking appears to protect from the development of sarcoidosis (and predisposes to the reactivation of TB), suggesting a destabilising effect of smoking on granuloma formation.

.2   **E: FEV$_1$ of 1.6**

To be a candidate for potentially curative surgery, there should be no evidence of metastatic spread, local invasion into other thoracic organs and no lymph node involvement beyond N1 (hilar nodes). By CT criteria, lymph nodes greater than 1 cubic centimetre are considered malignant until proven otherwise. Paraneoplastic phenomena (such as clubbing, HPOA, endocrinological disorders such as hypercalcaemia (caused by release of PTH-related peptide (PTH rp)) are not contraindications. There are also practical considerations to ensure a patient can successfully be taken off a ventilator postoperatively. In general, British Thoracic Society (BTS) guidelines recommend preoperative FEV$_1$ of greater that 1.5 (for lobectomy) and 2 (for pneumonectomy). In exceptional cases, patients with worse lung function can be considered after extensive physiological work-up (such as exercise testing, V/Q scanning).

.3   **E: Being the oldest sibling within a large family**

Current epidemiological data support the 'hygiene hypothesis'. Namely that the more Th1 stimulation the immune system receives during early childhood (through exposure to bacterial, mycobacterial and viral infections), the less likely it is to be inappropriately skewed towards a Th2 response to allergen. Conversely the more sterile an environment a young child is exposed to (developed country, urban living, obsessive new parents), the higher the chances of development of asthma.

3.4   C: Chest heaviness, fevers but no wheeze in the evenings

Questions on extrinsic allergic alveolitis (EAA) are particularly common. The condition is not an allergy (there is not a Th2 immune response associated with high IgE levels and eosinophilia and no associated wheeze). It is an immune complex (type III) and cell-mediated (type IV) hypersensitivity reaction triggered by a large number of organic particles (between 1 and 5 μm in size). In the USA, it is known as hypersensitivity pneumonitis. Short-term high level antigen exposure leads to acute EAA and the development (4–8 hours later) of cough, chest heaviness, fevers and myalgias (but no wheeze) characterised histologically by pneumonitis and granuloma formation. Long-term low-grade exposure results in chronic, irreversible lung fibrosis. As with other granulomatous lung diseases such as sarcoidosis, smoking is protective.

3.5   A: He is at increased risk of tuberculosis

Silicosis is an inorganic inhalational lung disease cause by exposure to silica (seen most commonly in quartz mining). Although acute silicosis (leading to acute lung injury and silicoproteinosis after massive inhalation) is occasionally seen, the most common presentation is with chronic silicosis which develops after 5–10 years of exposure and is characterised by multiple small pulmonary nodules (occasional eggshell calcification of hilar lymph nodes) but no change in lung function. As with other pneumoconiosis, a proportion will go on to develop progressive massive fibrosis leading to destruction of lung tissue (resulting in apical fibrosis) and significant physiological impairment. Macrophages, having taken up silica, become disabled or 'constipated' and can no longer respond to mycobacteria. This leads to increased susceptibility to TB. Additional complex immunological dysregulation also increases likelihood of developing autoimmune disease (in addition to an increased risk of bronchogenic carcinoma).

3.6   E: Can occur in rheumatoid arthritis

Rheumatoid arthritis can lead to the development of a localised or systemic vasculitis and occasionally produces pulmonary haemorrhage. Polyarteritis nodosa (PAN) is a medium vessel vasculitis, which rarely affects the lung (occasionally causing pulmonary vessel aneurysms). Microscopic polyarteritis

Answers: Respiratory Medicine

in contrast, is a recognised cause of pulmonary vasculitis and haemorrhage. TLCO and KCO are measures of lung absorbance of inhaled carbon monoxide (CO), which normally occurs when CO successfully diffuses from alveoli to capillaries and binds haemoglobin within red cells. In pulmonary haemorrhage, free haemoglobin within alveoli can efficiently absorb high TLCO and KCO values in these patients, despite huge V/Q mismatches, hypoxia and impaired oxygen delivery to capillaries.

.7   **A: Absence of vas deferens would make cystic fibrosis the most likely diagnosis**

There is an increasing number of young adults with recurrent chest infections and bronchiectasis that have been found to have mutations in the cystic fibrosis (CF) transmembrane regulator (CFTR) protein and have an atypical form of cystic fibrosis. These are not generally associated with homozygosity of the common CFTR mutation ΔF508 but rather with rarer mutations. Indeed, cases of isolated absence of vas deferens or pancreatic dysfunction (both typical of CF) with mutations in CFTR have been reported (and have normal lungs). Primary ciliary dyskinesia is associated with random embryological assignment of sidedness. So about 50% will have situs inversus and be classified as Kartagener's syndrome (situs inversus, otitis media, sinusitis, bronchiectasis and subfertility). Although recurrent pseudomonas infection may be caused by an immunodeficiency, it is commonly seen in conditions of impaired muco-ciliary clearance (as seen in CF).

.8   **D: His haemoglobin is 15 g/dl**

This question deals with compensation to high altitude and the subject of oxygen content of blood. Faced with chronic hypoxia, there is an increase in the red cell metabolite 2,3-DPG, which leads to decreased Hb affinity for O_2. This causes a right shift in the oxygen dissociation curve and more effective release of O_2 at the tissues. The main compensation to living at high altitude, however, is an increase in Hb (to about 20 g/dl), normalising the oxygen content of blood despite $p(O_2)$ of 6.1 and saturations of 81%. Oxygen delivery to tissues in this population is near normal.

.9   **D: Obesity**

Obesity is a well recognised cause of extra-thoracic restriction and predisposes to the development of chronic hypercapnia through hypoventilation. The four causes of obstructive spirometry are asthma, COPD (emphysema and chronic bronchitis), bronchiectasis and obliterative bronchiolitis. Simple coal worker pneumoconiosis, by definition, does not affect lung function.

3.10   A: Cerebral abscess

The lung has an important role in filtering out bacterial contaminants returning to the right side of the heart via the inferior vena cava (IVC). Bypassing this process, through a pulmonary AVM, increases likelihood of septic emboli and abscess development. Cerebral abscess is a significant cause of morbidity and mortality in patients with pulmonary AVMs

3.11   C: Respiratory rate of 35/min

The BTS guidelines on CAP (2004) highlight CURB-65 score as a useful prognostic indicator. The presence of: new onset **c**onfusion, **u**rea > 7, **r**espiratory rate > 30, hypotension (**B**P systolic < 90, diastolic < or = 60) and age > or = 65 are all core adverse prognostic factors.

3.12   D: V/Q highest at apex

As one moves from lung base to apex, perfusion falls (harder for blood to be pumped 'up hill'). Ventilation also falls but less steeply leading to an increasing V/Q ratio. The reason why ventilation falls is because in preinspiration, alveoli are squashed at the bases and expand during inspiration resulting in a large change in alveolar volume (and hence ventilation), while apical alveoli are already expanded preinspiration and undergo less change in volume during inspiration. On exercise, V/Q matching increases, due in part to collateral vessels opening up.

3.13   B: Are usually visible on bronchoscopy

Carcinoid tumours are highly vascular (and as a consequence appear as cherry red masses on bronchoscopy), predominantly occur in the central airways, rarely (<3%) produce symptoms of carcinoid syndrome and rarely (<10%) recur after surgical resection (which is usually curative). There is no association with smoking.

3.14   C: Occurs in farmer's lung

Apical fibrosis is associated with: allergic bronchopulmonary aspergillosis, radiation treatment, tuberculosis, sarcoidosis, extrinsic allergic alveolitis, Langerhans' cell histiocytosis, progressive massive fibrosis, chronic histoplasmosis and ankylosing spondylitis. However it is seen in less than 5% of cases of the

Answers: Respiratory Medicine

latter; the most important respiratory complication is found to be extrathoracic restriction.

.15   D: Commonly complicates lung disease in cystic fibrosis

From their early teens, patients with cystic fibrosis (CF) have increased incidence of pneumothoraces, which are often recurrent. Smoking increases risk of a pneumothorax in men by 22 times (even without any evidence of smoking related lung damage). Adult lung limited Langerhans' cell histiocytosis is a disease of young adults caused by an immune response to tobacco smoke leading to cystic lung destruction and frequently presents with pneumothorax. Lung involvement can also occur as part of multi-organ Langerhans' cell histiocytosis, which affects bones, lymph nodes and posterior pituitary (leading to diabetes insipidus), which is associated with monoclonal expansion of Langerhans' cells and a worse prognosis. In the context of normal underlying lung parenchyma, asymptomatic pneumothorax (usually < 10–15%; less than 3 cm from chest wall on X-ray) can be managed conservatively – the patient can potentially be discharged with written instructions on what to do if becomes symptomatic (ie return immediately to hospital). Symptomatic spontaneous pneumothorax should be managed by two attempts at aspiration initially (which will remove the necessity for chest drain insertion in 60% of cases). If aspiration fails, then a chest drain should be inserted. Patients with underlying parenchymal lung disease rarely have asymptomatic pneumothorax (their precarious lung function is usually compromised by even a small pneumothorax). Admission is almost always warranted even if they are treated conservatively. Symptomatic pneumothoraces in this population group should be treated by chest drain insertion since aspiration almost inevitably fails. Patients involved in trauma (such as road traffic accidents) should have chest drains inserted for all pneumothoraces (as per *ATLS Guidelines*).

.16   B: Improvement occurs following treatment with prednisolone and oral itraconazole

Allergic bronchopulmonary aspergillosis is associated with thick sputum plugs and exacerbation of asthma in susceptible patients. Peripheral blood eosinophilia and raised serum IgE and specific IgE are characteristic (measured skinprick by either skinprick testing or RAST testing). Chest X-ray/CT may show upper lobe infiltrates with proximal bronchiectasis. Precipitating antibodies (IgG) to *Aspergillus* antigen are also occasionally positive. Treatment is with steroids and oral itraconazole. Intravenous amphotericin (or newer antifungals such as voriconazole and caspofungin) are used to treat invasive aspergillosis, which occurs in the immunosuppressed. Controversy exists on the best

management for asymptomatic aspergilloma. Related haemoptysis require
treatment (either surgical resection or embolisation).

3.17   B: Chronic stable asthma

Carbon monoxide (CO) transfer factor measures gas transfer between alveo
and blood. Usually, a single breath of gas containing a known low concentra
tion of CO is taken, held for 10 seconds, then expired. Measurement of expire
gas volume and CO concentration enables calculation of CO uptake by bloo
flowing through pulmonary capillaries. When free blood is present in th
bronchial tree/alveoli (such as during pulmonary haemorrhage), transfer factc
is high as the haemoglobin binds the CO (also high in polycythaemia). Ga
transfer may be high in chronic stable asthmatics for a number of reason:
hyperexpansion (as a consequence of gas trapping), in the absence of signif
cant parenchymal damage, can increase available surface area for gas ex
change; additionally the cardiac output may be increased compared to health
controls, which optimises V/Q matching. In contrast, CO absorbance
reduced in patients with emphysema dueto destruction of gas exchangin
surface and mismatching of ventilation and perfusion.

3.18   C: Flow/volume loop

PEFR and the FEV_1 to FVC ratio will be low in both asthma and upper airway
obstruction. The two tests together may be useful, since in upper airway
obstruction PEFR is usually (but not always) disproportionately reduced com
pared with FEV_1. The FEV_1 (ml) divided by PEFR (l/min) is usually less than 10
Values greater than 10 are very suggestive of large airways obstructio
Inspection of typical flow/volume loops, the best physiological test for distin
guishing asthma from upper airways obstruction, will help explain why this
the case.

3.19   E: Tuberculous meningitis co-exists in 15–20% of patients

Miliary tuberculosis is defined as progressive, haematologically disseminate
Mycobacterium TB infection. This occurs as a result of failed cell mediate
immunity. The tuberculin test is usually negative. The classic radiograph
picture of multiple millet seed-size (1–2 mm) pulmonary lesions gives th
condition its name but the chest X-ray may be normal for months befo
development of miliary shadows. Indeed, up to one-third of chest X-rays a
normal. On presentation patients, particularly the elderly, may be mild
unwell with only unexplained anaemia or fever for long periods before dia
nosis. Hyponatraemia is well recognised (as result of SIADH). Approximate

Answers: Respiratory Medicine

15–20% of adults with miliary tuberculosis have tuberculous meningitis at the time of presentation and about one-third of patients with TB meningitis have concomitant miliary TB.

.20   C: Difficulty in getting to sleep at night

The systemic hypertension often seen in patients with obstructive sleep apnoea (OSA) is poorly understood but is reduced by treating the OSA. Pulmonary hypertension and secondary polycythaemia are thought to result from the hypoxaemia that accompanies the episodes of apnoea, and which in some individuals may persist during waking hours. Daytime somnolence is characteristic; patients may fall asleep while driving, eating or talking. Depression affects at least 25% of patients.

.21   D: Hypertrophic pulmonary osteoarthropathy (HPOA) can resolve if the primary tumour is treated

Small-cell carcinoma has a short doubling time of 30 days and has usually spread by the time of presentation. Combination chemotherapy with agents such as cyclophosphamide, vincristine, etoposide, adriamycin and methotrexate have been tried. Studies have suggested that six cycles of treatment at 3- to 4-week intervals is optimal. No survival advantage was noted in having further courses or maintenance chemotherapy. Adriamycin is cardiotoxic. Vinca alkaloids such as vincristine cause demyelination leading to peripheral neuropathy. Most cytotoxic agents are myelotoxic. Cisplatin is nephrotoxic and can also cause a sensory peripheral neuropathy and tinnitus. HPOA is rare in small-cell lung carcinoma and commonest in squamous cell carcinoma. It is associated with finger clubbing in 90% of cases.

.22   B: Eaton–Lambert syndrome occurs most commonly with small-cell carcinoma

Progressive proximal muscle weakness and dysphagia are characteristic of Eaton–Lambert syndrome. EMG reveals post-tetanic potentiation and muscles get stronger with repeat contraction. The syndrome is caused by antibodies against presynaptic calcium channels. So increasing action potential frequency can overcome this block of neuromuscular junction transmission. The presence of SIADH results in a dilutional hyponatraemia, low plasma osmolality (less than 260 mOsmol/kg) and a high urine osmolality. Treatment is with demeclocycline that causes a nephrogenic diabetes insipidus by competing for ADH at the renal tubule. In this context, SIADH is almost always associated with small-cell lung carcinoma and will improve following chemotherapy. The commonest cause of hypercalcaemia is not bony metastases, rather tumour secretion o PTH-related peptide (PTH-rp).

3.23   D: CT pulmonary angiogram (spiral CT) scanning

This patient has a high pre-test probability of having a pulmonary embolism (therefore D-dimer testing is not indicated). CT pulmonary angiogram scanning is the most appropriate investigation since it will almost always detect significant PE, assess clot burden and detect alternative respiratory diagnoses. In addition, there is significant intraobserver agreement and it does not require cardiological expertise (which is frequently unavailable in the acute setting).

3.24   D: Ipsilateral supraclavicular lymph node metastasis

Lung cancer is inoperable if: stage IIIB or worse; pleural effusion (if malignant aetiology); nerve entrapment (phrenic or recurrent laryngeal); superior vena cava (SVC) obstruction; distant metastases; or FEV_1 less than 1.0–1.5 litres. As far as TNM staging is concerned, any N2 or N3 (contralateral hilar o mediastinal nodes) or any T4 (any tumour of any size with invasion o mediastinum or involving heart, great vessels, trachea, oesophagus, vertebra body, carina or malignant pleural effusion) tumour is considered inoperable.

ANSWERS

Rheumatology and Immunology

RHEUMATOLOGY AND IMMUNOLOGY: 'BEST OF FIVE' ANSWERS

.1   E: Persistence of rheumatoid factor at high titre is a risk factor for the development of rheumatoid arthritis

Around 70% of all patients with established rheumatoid arthritis and up to 100% of patients with nodules are seropositive for IgM rheumatoid factor. However, the prevalence is much lower at disease onset and it is found in other connective tissue diseases, in response to infection (particularly chronic infection), and the prevalence is increased in the elderly (up to 30% in some series). Presence of rheumatoid factor is the best predictor of erosive outcome, identified to date, in rheumatoid arthritis. A persistently raised titre has been shown to increase the probability of developing rheumatoid arthritis in the future.

.2   A: Interstitial lung disease

Pulmonary involvement is the leading cause of death in diffuse systemic sclerosis and usually arises because of progressive fibrotic lung disease. Pulmonary hypertension does occur in some cases but less commonly than in the limited cutaneous form of the disease. Myocardial disease and arrhythmias are recognised causes of sudden death. Scleroderma renal crisis is characterised by accelerated hypertension, microangiopathic haemolysis and consumptive thrombocytopenia. It used to be the commonest cause of death but early introduction of angiotensin-converting enzyme (ACE) inhibitors has resulted in a dramatic improvement in rates of survival from this complication.

.3   A: If he is found to carry the HLA-B27 antigen the course is more likely to be chronic

The history is suggestive of reactive arthritis secondary to a dysenteric infection. The joint swelling is characteristically sterile and treatment with antibiotics will have no effect on the course of the arthritis. The classic triad is of arthritis, non-gonococcal urethritis and conjunctivitis, but conjunctivitis only occurs in approximately 30% of cases. The sacro-iliac joints may be involved and this can be unilateral or bilateral. HLA-B27 has prognostic implications because, if present, the arthritis is more likely to become chronic or recurrent.

.4   C: Dermatomyositis

The history is typical of dermatomyositis with skin involvement manifesting as the shawl sign, with a characteristic distribution involving the face, upper arms and neck. Although photosensitivity is characteristic of SLE, it also occurs in dermatomyositis. ANA is likely to be positive in many connective tissue diseases and therefore will not help in diagnosis. The absence of antibodies to RNP makes a diagnosis of mixed connective tissue disease unlikely, whilst the absence of sclerodactyly or thickened skin makes systemic sclerosis unlikely.

4.5   B: Lymphopenia

Differentiating a flare of lupus from super-imposed infection can be difficult but is important because management of the former may require a higher dose of steroids while the latter requires antibiotic treatment. Most inflammatory markers, including erythrocyte sedimentation rate (ESR) and GGT, will be elevated in both situations. However, the C-reactive protein (CRP) is usually normal in active lupus but elevated in infection. Complement components C4 and C3 are usually low in lupus flare and this is due to active consumption of these molecules. A leucopenia, particularly lymphopenia, with a normal bone marrow again occurs in active lupus but neutrophilia is more common with infection.

4.6   D: Polyarteritis nodosa (PAN)

Wegener's granulomatosis can affect the eyes, ENT and upper respiratory tract, lower respiratory tract and kidneys, and involve the peripheral or central nervous systems. However, vasculitis involving the gastrointestinal tract is uncommon. Microscopic polyangiitis primarily affects the kidneys and Churg–Strauss syndrome is associated with atopy, peripheral neuropathy, eosinophilia and fleeting pulmonary granuloma. Both Henoch–Schönlein vasculitis and PAN can involve the gastrointestinal tract, kidneys and skin but PAN is more commonly associated with a peripheral neuropathy. Henoch–Schönlein vasculitis can occur in adults but is much commoner in children.

4.7   E: Rectal biopsy

The most likely diagnosis is amyloid, resulting from long-standing poorly controlled inflammation. The fibrils consist of AA amyloid as opposed to AL amyloid, which occurs in monoclonal gammopathies (cardiac involvement more likely with this form of amyloidosis). The commonest presentation is with renal abnormalities, which can range from mild proteinuria to frank nephritic syndrome. A total of 80% cases will be picked up on rectal biopsy (subcutaneous fat aspiration can also be performed) and there is characteristic staining with congo red on polarising light microscopy.

Answers: Rheumatology and Immunology

8.8   C: Osteoarthritis (OA) is the most likely diagnosis

Hyperuricaemia is ten times more common than gout and uric acid levels can be normal during a flare-up of gout. Hence, uric acid can neither confirm nor exclude a diagnosis of gout in this case where joint pain is current. Similarly, chondrocalcinosis (presence of calcium in the joint) is much more common than pseudogout and the commonest joints involved are the knees, wrists and index metacarpal joints (haemochromatosis). Osteoarthritis commonly affects the first MTP joint and, until the diagnosis is confirmed, treatment with allopurinol should not be commenced. In the absence of a positive family history, a history of alcohol excess or other medication, OA is more likely than gout.

8.9   B: Erythrocyte sedimentation rate (ESR)

In this age group, polymyalgia rheumatica (PMR) is much more likely than myositis as a cause of difficulty lifting the arms above the head. Movement is restricted due to stiffness in PMR as opposed to weakness in myositis. Muscle biopsies and creatinine kinase can be normal in myositis, particularly dermato-myositis. While the ESR will be high in myositis, it will be very high in PMR and, therefore, this is the best test.

8.10   E: Osteoporosis is diagnosed when the T score is ⩽ −2.5

Not all treatments are effective in all patients, so it is wise to obtain baseline bone density readings to enable you to monitor the effectiveness of the osteoprotection. Etidronate is used as prophylaxis for steroid-induced osteoporosis but is complicated to take and may not be the best choice for an elderly woman. All trials of bisphosphonates have used calcium supplementation and, especially as this woman is immobile and elderly, there may be some co-existing osteomalacia. Results of bone density scanning should be compared to the peak bone mass (T score) rather than to an age-matched control (Z score).

8.11   C: Angiotensin-converting enzyme (ACE) inhibitors should be introduced as soon as any rise in blood pressure is noted

The fact that this woman has tight skin, which includes her upper arms, indicates that she has diffuse systemic sclerosis (dSSc) rather than limited cutaneous (lcSSc), where skin involvement is limited to the hands and forearms, the head and neck and the legs and feet. Trials of penicillamine in treating the skin changes of systemic sclerosis have been disappointing. The commonest cause of death in dSSc is pulmonary fibrosis. Pulmonary hypertension does occur in around 5% of cases but is more common as a late complication of lcSSc (CREST) (~25% cases). ANA may be positive in many connective tissue diseases. A serious complication of dSSc is scleroderma renal crisis, which is associated with renal failure and death. The introduction of ACE inhibitors at an early stage can preserve renal function and avert this complication.

4.12   C: Oligoarthritis affecting the lower limbs, associated with bilateral hilar lymphadenopathy and erythema nodosum

The most common form of joint involvement in sarcoidosis is an arthropathy affecting particularly the large joints of the lower limb, often associated with bilateral hilar lymphadenopathy, erythema nodosum, uveitis or lupus pernio. The joints are affected in a symmetrical manner and the arthropathy can last for weeks to months. Erythema chronicum migrans is characteristic of Lyme disease.

4.13   B: Arthritis of the distal interphalangeal (DIP) joints is usually associated with nail involvement

Psoriatic arthritis (PsA) is an inflammatory arthritis associated with psoriasis and usually negative for rheumatoid factor. However, the presence of rheumatoid factor (RF) does not exclude the diagnosis. The commonest presentation is with an oligoarthritis affecting the large joints of the lower limbs but DIP joint involvement is the classic presentation and is almost always associated with nail involvement. The prevalence of HLA-B27 is higher in PsA, particularly in those with sacro-iliac joint involvement. However, HLA-B27 is also found in the normal population and cannot, therefore, be used to confirm the diagnosis. There is a risk of antimalarials exacerbating skin psoriasis but they can be used to treat the arthritis. Acute anterior uveitis is the characteristic ocular manifestation.

4.14   B: *Staphylococcus aureus*

Staphylococcus aureus accounts for over 50% of infection and β-haemolytic *Streptococcus* around 10%. In children under 2 years of age *Haemophilus* is common. Lower limbs tend to be affected more than upper limbs. In children the commonest site is the hips while the knee is involved more often in adults. *Neisseria gonorrhoeae* is a cause of septic arthritis in young adults and is often associated with painless skin lesions. Lyme disease is caused by the spirochaet *Borrelia burgdorferi*. It presents with erythema marginatum at the site of the tick bite, arthritis (recurrent brief attacks), neurological (lymphocytic meningitis encephalomyelitis) and cardiac (second-/third-degree arteriovenous (AV) conduction defects) complications.

4.15   C: Chronic anterior iridocyclitis

The iris and ciliary body both form the anterior uveal tract. Therefore, iridocyclitis is anterior uveitis. Chronic asymptomatic anterior uveitis is a well-recognised complication of juvenile idiopathic arthritis, particular the pauciarticular forms. It is bilateral in two-thirds of cases and therefore regular slit lamp screening examinations are required as it may lead to blindness. Acute anterior uveitis is characteristic of the seronegative spondyloarthropathies, while conjunctivitis occurs in Reiter's/reactive arthritis. Scleritis occurs in rheumatoid arthritis, SLE, Wegener's granulomatosis and other forms of vasculitis. Posterior uveitis occurs in Behçet's disease, Wegener's granulomatosis and sarcoidosis.

4.16   E: Any of these items

Non-steroidal anti-inflammatory drugs (NSAIDs) may interact with a number of different medications. Methotrexate and lithium levels may rise. Although a recognised interaction, it is very common to find patients on both methotrexate and an NSAID. Monitoring of the full blood count and liver function every 4 to 6 weeks is essential with methotrexate treatment, whether taking NSAIDs or not. The effectiveness of thiazides, loop diuretics, β-blockers, angiotensin-converting enzyme (ACE) inhibitors and oral hypoglycaemic agents may fall. There is also an increased risk of hyperkalaemia with potassium-sparing diuretics. The patient is also taking corticosteroids. This may increase the risk of gastrointestinal bleeding and exacerbate fluid retention.

4.17   C: Use of a β-blocker

Men over the age of 60 years may lose bone density, but the risk of osteoporotic fracture does not appear to increase in men until after the age of 70. Other risk factors include hypogonadism (low testosterone levels), smoking, chronic alcohol abuse, lack of exercise, poor nutrition, drugs (such as corticosteroids, heparin, thyroxine and phenytoin) and disorders such as rheumatoid arthritis, diabetes mellitus, chronic liver or renal disease, malabsorption syndromes and endocrinopathies (Cushing's syndrome, hyperthyroidism, hyperparathyroidism). Low-trauma fractures should be investigated with dual energy X-ray absorptiometry (DEXA) at all ages, though there is an argument for commencing the elderly patient (>80 years) on calcium and vitamin D without scanning and/or newer bisphosphonates in the presence of new spinal fractures.

4.18   C: Drugs implicated in the aetiology of DIL should not be used in idiopathic systemic lupus erythematosus

Many drugs have been implicated in causing drug-induced lupus (DIL) and i often arises as a side-effect of long-term use of certain medications. Specific criteria for diagnosing DIL have not been formally established. However, some symptoms overlap with those of SLE. These include:

- muscle and joint pain and swelling
- flu-like symptoms of fatigue and fever
- serositis (inflammation around the lungs or heart that causes pain o discomfort)
- ANA positive.

Those drugs definitely and most commonly associated with DIL are hydrala zine, procainamide, isoniazid, quinidine, methyldopa, chlorpromazine and salazopyrin. Hydralazine associated DIL is considered to be dose-dependen and procainamide time dependent. Up to 90% of patients taking procainamide develop a positive antinuclear antibody (ANA) and 30% of these develop DIL Renal, central nervous system and skin features of SLE are rare in DIL. Othe features of SLE, such as articular, pulmonary and serosal disease are common In the majority of cases the condition subsides on withdrawing the drug. There is no contraindication to using these drugs in idiopathic SLE.

4.19   E: All of the options

The granular, diffuse and cytoplasm-distributed c-ANCA affects the targe antigen proteinase 3 and is associated with Wegener's granulomatosis. The perinuclear distributed p-ANCA binds to several enzymes, including myeloper oxidase and is associated with microscopic polyangiitis, polyarteritis nodosa Churg–Strauss syndrome, Felty's syndrome and inflammatory bowel disease An atypical perinuclear a-ANCA is found in inflammatory bowel diseases endocarditis and HIV.

4.20   D: Elevated C-reactive protein (CRP) and a normochromic normocytic anaemia

An abnormal muscle biopsy, an abnormal EMG and high signal intensity seer on T2-weighted MRI scans of the thighs are all characteristic of polymyositis rather than polymyalgia rheumatica (PMR). Both present with symptoms affect ing the proximal limb girdle muscles but polymyositis characteristically pre sents with weakness where as the predominant symptom in PMR is join stiffness. All acute phase proteins (including ESR, CRP, antitrypsin orosomucoic and haptoglobin) are elevated in PMR. As with any chronic inflammation, the

Answers: Rheumatology and Immunology

anaemia of chronic disease is common. Although 15% patients with PMR have co-existing temporal arteritis, the presence of skip lesions is not characteristic of PMR itself.

4.21   D: Atlanto-axial subluxation

The commonest complication of ankylosing spondylitis (AS) is acute (not chronic) anterior uveitis, which affects 25–30% at some point in the disease course. It is usually unilateral and associated with the presence of the HLA-B27 antigen. Approximately 10% of cases develop cardiac complications including aortic incompetence, aortitis and AV conduction abnormalities. These complications become more common with increasing disease duration and are commoner in those with peripheral as well as axial joint disease. Apical lung fibrosis tends to be associated with long disease duration (~20 years). It is bilateral in most cases and presents with cough, shortness of breath and occasionally with haemoptysis. Approximately 2% of patients with AS develop atlanto-axial subluxation. This complication is more frequent in patients with rheumatoid arthritis (RA) but in both conditions can present with quadriplegia. Other rare complications of long-standing AS include amyloid and IgA nephropathy.

4.22   A: Systemic lupus erythematosus

The X-ray findings typical of rheumatoid arthritis are periarticular osteopenia, juxta-articular bony erosions, subluxation and bony deformity. The proximal interphalangeal (PIPJ) and the metacarpophalangeal joints (MCPJ) are affected. Lupus arthritis is non-erosive. Up to 10% of patients with lupus arthritis will develop reversible deformities of the hands and feet associated with weakening of cartilage and bone (Jaccoud-type deformities). In osteoarthritis, the first carpometacarpal (CMCJ) and the distal interphalangeal joints (DIPJ) are more commonly affected. Joint space narrowing, osteophyte formation and subchondral sclerosis are seen. In psoriatic arthritis, the DIPJ as well as the PIPJ and MCPJ can be involved. The pattern is characteristically asymmetrical. Classic X-ray changes include 'pencil-in-cup' deformities and ankylosis (fusion of bones across a joint). The classical radiographic sign of gout is osseous erosions, manifested as 'punched-out' lesions at the margins of the articular surfaces of the hands and feet; these erosions contain sclerotic borders and are classically associated with over-hanging edges. The pattern of joint involvement shows asymmetry and the 1st MTPJ is often involved.

4.23   D: Systemic lupus erythematosus

Autoantibodies to dsDNA are found in up to 60% of cases of systemic lupus erythematosus (SLE). The antibody is associated with nephritis and severe disease. The Sm autoantibody is found in up to 40% of cases and associated with interstitial lung disease. It is very uncommon to find these autoantibodies in association with other autoimmune rheumatic diseases. Autoantibodies to snRNP are also common in SLE, but are less specific and may be found in overlap syndromes with features of polymyositis and systemic sclerosis. Anti-Ro and anti-La antibodies may be found in 10–30% of SLE patients. They are, however, more commonly associated with Sjögren's syndrome. Less than 5% of patients with SLE will have Scl-70 autoantibodies (indicative of diffuse systemic sclerosis), centromere autoantibodies (indicative of limited scleroderma) or Jo-1 autoantibodies (suggestive of poly-/dermatomyositis).

4.24   E: All of the options

All of the options are associated with aggressive disease in rheumatoid arthritis. Other features include an elevated ESR, bony erosions on plain X-rays and multiple joint involvement.

4.25   E: Start the patient on 60 mg/day oral prednisolone

Temporal arteritis, often associated with polymyalgia rheumatica, tends to occur abruptly and is commonly associated with either a temporal or occipital headache, scalp tenderness, constitutional symptoms, jaw claudication and visual disturbance. In the presence of the latter, high-dose oral prednisolone should be commenced immediately to try to prevent visual loss from ischaemic optic neuropathy. A high erythrocyte sedimentation rate (ESR) and histological evidence of arteritis are useful diagnostic tests. Although a biopsy is best performed as early as possible, the introduction of prednisolone should never be delayed. The dose of steroid can be tapered downwards slowly in steps of 5–10 mg every 2 to 4 weeks according to symptom control and a falling ESR. When the daily dose has reached 10 mg/day it is advised that a slower tapering regime be employed at 1-mg reductions every two weeks. Most patients will require daily maintenance doses of approximately 5 mg for 12 to 24 months. Some cases require longer-term and higher-dose maintenance therapy. In cases where this seems likely (prednisolone dose ≥ 7.5 mg/day for 3 months), prophylaxis against corticosteroid-induced osteoporosis should be started.

Answers: Rheumatology and Immunology

4.26   D: Measure spirochaete antibodies

Lyme disease (LD) is a spirochaete (*Borrelia burgdorferi*) tick-borne infection common throughout the world and in particular northern USA. The hallmark of LD is an annular erythematous and often large (> 20 cm) rash (erythema chronicum migrans (ECM)) at the site of the tick bite. However, many people do not recall the bite or the rash. Constitutional symptoms of fever and fatigue may precede headaches, myalgia, arthralgia, tendonopathy, conjunctivitis, uveitis, pharyngitis, lymphadenopathy and testicular swelling. Weeks later there may be cardiac or neurological symptoms and months later there may be a persistent inflammatory arthropathy and an atrophic rash of acrodermatitis chronica atrophicans. Raised IgG or specific IgM antibodies to the spirochaete can be found 2 to 4 weeks after infection. The diagnosis is clinical, supported by this serological test. Early disease is best treated with amoxicillin, doxycycline or clarithromycin. Later cardiac, neurological or persistent arthritic symptoms may also require a cephalosporin.

4.27   E: Warfarin should be dosed to maintain the INR at 2.0

Antiphospholipid syndrome is associated with recurrent venous and arterial thrombosis, spontaneous abortion, vasculitis, central nervous system (CNS) disorders and a 'catastrophic' widespread organ failure. Thrombocytopenia is seen in up to 25% of cases. Antibodies are found in 5% of the general population and in association with several autoimmune rheumatic diseases (especially SLE), vasculitides, infection and malignancy. Both the lupus anticoagulant and anticardiolipin antibodies should be measured though one and not the other may be present in up to 40% of cases. The lupus anticoagulant cannot be measured if the patient is already on heparin or warfarin. Recurrent thrombosis should be treated with high-dose warfarin at an INR of 3–4.

4.28   A: Dermatomyositis

The following are recognised causes of ectopic calcification: hyperparathyroidism, hyperphosphataemia, sarcoidosis, hypervitaminosis D, tumour lysis, dermatomyositis, scleroderma.

4.29   E: Is associated with acute anterior uveitis independently of systemic joint disease

HLA-B27 is a normal gene variant found in 8% of the White population and only 2% of people with this variant will eventually get spondylitis. Hence, the HLA-B27 test is not diagnostic of ankylosing spondylitis (AS). The association between AS and HLA-B27 varies in different ethnic and racial groups: the frequency of the variant in patients with AS is over 95% in White patients, 80% in Mediterranean populations and 50% in African-American patients with AS. Osteitis condensans ilii is a benign condition typically seen after pregnancy and can be confused with ankylosing spondylitis as the sacro-iliac joints can be affected in a symmetrical manner. Symmetrical triangular shaped sclerosis occurs around the lower part of the sacro-iliac joints, mainly affecting the iliac side of the sacro-iliac joints but there is no evidence of narrowing or irregularity in the joint space on both sides. No association exists with HLA-B27. HLA-B27 is associated with acute anterior uveitis even in the absence of systemic disease.

4.30   E: Raised parathyroid hormone

Pseudohypoparathyroidism (PHP) occurs as a result of target tissue resistance to parathyroid hormone (PTH). The biochemical consequences are hypocalcaemia, hyperphosphataemia and a raised PTH. Pseudohypoparathyroidism may be tested for by measuring urine excretion of cyclic AMP (cAMP) in response to PTH. Administration of parathyroid hormone (PTH) to normal individuals leads to increased urinary excretion of cAMP. An abnormal response to this test in individuals with PHP classifies them as either type I (no increase in urine cAMP) or type II (normal increase in urine cAMP but abnormal renal phosphate handling). The clinical features of PHT include short stature, round facies, obesity and brachydactyly. Pseudopseudohypoparathyroidism describes the clinical features in the presence of a normal serum calcium and PTH/cAMP test.

REVISION CHECKLISTS

CARDIOLOGY: REVISION CHECKLIST

Valvular heart disease

❏ Heart sounds
❏ Mitral stenosis
❏ Valve lesions/murmurs
❏ Antibiotic prophylaxis
❏ Catheterisation data
❏ Mitral valve prolapse
❏ Infective endocarditis

Arrhythmias

❏ Wolff–Parkinson–White/SVT
❏ Atrial fibrillation
❏ Ventricular tachycardia
❏ LBBB
❏ Prolonged QT interval
❏ Torsades de pointes
❏ Indications for pacing

Pericardial and myocardial disease

❏ Constrictive pericarditis
❏ Cardiac tamponade
❏ Pericardial effusion
❏ IHD/heart muscle disease
❏ Myocardial infarction
❏ Cardiomyopathy
❏ Left ventricular failure
❏ Unstable angina
❏ Coronary bypass surgery/Angioplasty
❏ Left ventricular hypertrophy
❏ Signs underlying heart disease

Congenital heart disease

☐ Cyanotic heart disease/Eisenmenger's

☐ ASD

☐ Patent ductus arteriosus

☐ VSD

Large vessel disease

☐ Pulmonary embolus

☐ Aortic dissection

☐ Pulmonary hypertension

Miscellaneous

☐ Cannon *a* waves in JVP

☐ Alcohol and the heart

☐ Carotid body/cardiac sympathetics

☐ Coronary circulation

☐ Left atrial myxoma

☐ Hypertension

HAEMATOLOGY: REVISION CHECKLIST

Red cell physiology and anaemias

- ❏ Iron deficiency/metabolism/therapy
- ❏ Macrocytosis/pernicious anaemia
- ❏ Folate deficiency
- ❏ Basophilia
- ❏ Erythropoiesis/haemoglobin physiology
- ❏ Haem biosynthesis
- ❏ Sideroblastic anaemia
- ❏ Aplastic anaemia
- ❏ Investigation of anaemia
- ❏ Vitamin B12 metabolism

Haemolytic anaemia

- ❏ Haemolytic anaemia
- ❏ Sickle cell/haemoglobinopathy
- ❏ Hereditary spherocytosis
- ❏ Reticulocytosis
- ❏ G6PD deficiency
- ❏ Haemolytic–uraemic syndrome
- ❏ Thrombotic thrombocytopaenic purpura
- ❏ Intravascular haemolysis

Bleeding disorders

- ❏ Thrombocytopenia
- ❏ Haemophilia
- ❏ Coagulation cascade
- ❏ Fresh-frozen plasma
- ❏ von Willebrand's disease
- ❏ Warfarin/Vitamin K/Clotting Pathway

Haematological malignancy

- ☐ Hodgkin's/non-Hodgkin's lymphoma
- ☐ Leukaemia
- ☐ Pancytopenia/splenomegaly
- ☐ Polycythaemia

Miscellaneous

- ☐ Hyposplenism
- ☐ Methaemoglobinaemia
- ☐ Neutropenia
- ☐ Thrombocytosis
- ☐ Bone infarction
- ☐ Bone marrow test
- ☐ Eosinophilia
- ☐ Hyperuricaemia and haematological disease
- ☐ Paroxysmal nocturnal haemoglobinuria

RESPIRATORY MEDICINE: REVISION CHECKLIST

Respiratory infections

❏ Pneumonia

❏ Bronchopulmonary aspergillosis

❏ Acute bronchiolitis

❏ Psittacosis

❏ Viral infections

❏ TB

Lung cancer

❏ Bronchial carcinoma

❏ Surgery for cancer

❏ Pancoast's tumour

❏ Small-cell cancer

❏ Mesothelioma

Pulmonary physiology

❏ Anatomy of the lung

❏ Lung function tests

❏ Normal physiology

❏ Transfer factor

❏ Forced hyperventilation

End-stage lung disease

❏ Respiratory failure

❏ Long-term oxygen

Interstitial lung disease/fibrosis

- ☐ Extrinsic allergic alveolitis
- ☐ Bronchiectasis
- ☐ ARDS
- ☐ Sarcoidosis
- ☐ Emphysema
- ☐ Fibrosing alveolitis
- ☐ Pulmonary fibrosis
- ☐ Asbestosis
- ☐ Cystic fibrosis

Miscellaneous

- ☐ Asthma
- ☐ Sleep-apnoea syndrome
- ☐ Autoimmune disease and the lung
- ☐ Abnormal chest X-ray
- ☐ Lung cavitation
- ☐ Pulmonary eosinophilia
- ☐ Pleural effusion

RHEUMATOLOGY: REVISION CHECKLIST

Autoimmune disease

❏ Rheumatoid arthritis

❏ SLE

❏ Wegener's granulomatosis

Other vasculitides

❏ Polymyalgia rheumatica

❏ Cranial arteritis

❏ Vasculitic disease

Other arthritides

❏ Reiter's syndrome

❏ Ankylosing spondylitis/HLA-B27

❏ Arthralgia

❏ Behçet's disease

❏ Arthropathy (general)

❏ Hypertrophic osteoarthropathy

❏ Osteoarthritis

❏ Pseudogout

Miscellaneous

❏ Antiphospholipid syndrome

❏ Digital gangrene

❏ Peri-articular calcification

❏ Systemic sclerosis

IMMUNOLOGY: REVISION CHECKLIST

Cytokines
- ☐ Tumour necrosis factor
- ☐ Interferon
- ☐ Inflammatory mediators (general)
- ☐ Leukotrienes

Cellular immunity
- ☐ T lymphocytes/deficiency
- ☐ Cell-mediated immunity

Immunoglobulins/autoimmunity
- ☐ IgA/IgE/IgG
- ☐ Autoimmune disease/ANCA
- ☐ Hypogammaglobulinaemia
- ☐ Monoclonal gammopathy
- ☐ Tissue receptor antibodies
- ☐ Circulating immune complexes
- ☐ Precipitating antibodies in diagnosis

Miscellaneous
- ☐ Complement/CH50
- ☐ Angioneurotic oedema
- ☐ Hypersensitivity reactions
- ☐ Mast cells
- ☐ Polymerase chain reaction
- ☐ Post-splenectomy
- ☐ Transplant rejection
- ☐ Acute phase reactants

INDEX

Index

HAEMATOLOGY

Index

RESPIRATORY MEDICINE

RHEUMATOLOGY